Assessment of Exposure-Response Functions for Rocket-Emission Toxicants

Subcommittee on Rocket-Emission Toxicants
Committee on Toxicology
Board on Environmental Studies and Toxicology
Commission on Life Sciences
National Research Council

NATIONAL ACADEMY PRESS
Washington, D.C. 1998

NATIONAL ACADEMY PRESS   2101 Constitution Ave., N.W.   Washington, D.C. 20418

NOTICE: The project that is the subject of this report was approved by the Governing Board of the National Research Council, whose members are drawn from the councils of the National Academy of Sciences, the National Academy of Engineering, and the Institute of Medicine. The members of the committee responsible for the report were chosen for their special competences and with regard for appropriate balance.

This report has been reviewed by a group other than the authors according to procedures approved by a Report Review Committee consisting of members of the National Academy of Sciences, the National Academy of Engineering, and the Institute of Medicine.

This project was supported by Contract No. DAMD 17-89-C-9086 between the National Academy of Sciences and the U.S. Department of Defense. Any opinions, findings, conclusions, or recommendations expressed in this publication are those of the author(s) and do not necessarily reflect the view of the organizations or agencies that provided support for this project.

Library of Congress Catalog Card Number 98-86245
International Standard Book Number 0-309-06144-X

Additional copies of this report are available from:

National Academy Press
2101 Constitution Ave., NW
Box 285
Washington, DC 20055
800-624-6242
202-334-3313 (in the Washington metropolitan area)
http://www.nap.edu

Copyright 1998 by the National Academy of Sciences. All rights reserved.

Printed in the United States of America

SUBCOMMITTEE ON ROCKET-EMISSION TOXICANTS

DONALD E. GARDNER *(Chair)*, Inhalation Toxicology Associates, Raleigh, N.C.
CHARLES E. FEIGLEY, University of South Carolina School of Public Health, Columbia, S.C.
DAVID W. GAYLOR, U.S. Food and Drug Administration, Jefferson, Ark.
THOMAS E. MCKONE, University of California School of Public Health and Lawrence Berkeley National Laboratory, Berkeley, Calif.
JOHN L. O'DONOGHUE, Eastman Kodak Company, Rochester, N.Y.
HANSPETER R. WITSCHI, University of California, Davis, Calif.
GAROLD S. YOST, University of Utah, Salt Lake City, Utah

Staff

KULBIR S. BAKSHI, Program Director for the Committee on Toxicology
CAROL A. MACZKA, Study Director
MARGARET E. MCVEY, Staff Officer
RUTH E. CROSSGROVE, Editor
CATHERINE M. KUBIK, Senior Program Assistant
LINDA V. LEONARD, Senior Project Assistant
LUCY V. FUSCO, Project Assistant

Sponsor

U.S. Department of Defense

COMMITTEE ON TOXICOLOGY

ROGENE F. HENDERSON *(Chair)*, Lovelace Biomedical and Environmental Research Institute, Albuquerque, N.Mex.
DONALD E. GARDNER *(Vice-Chair)*, Inhalation Toxicology Associates, Raleigh, N.C.
GERMAINE M. BUCK, State University at Buffalo, Buffalo, N.Y.
GARY P. CARLSON, Purdue University, West Lafayette, Ind.
JACK H. DEAN, Sanofi Winthrop, Inc., Malvern, Pa.
KEVIN E. DRISCOLL, The Procter & Gamble Co., Cincinnati, Ohio
ELAINE M. FAUSTMAN, University of Washington, Seattle, Wash.
CHARLES E. FEIGLEY, University of South Carolina School of Public Health, Columbia, S.C.
DAVID W. GAYLOR, U.S. Food and Drug Administration, Jefferson, Ark.
JUDITH A. GRAHAM, U.S. Environmental Protection Agency, Research Triangle Park, N.C.
IAN A. GREAVES, University of Minnesota, Minneapolis, Minn.
SIDNEY GREEN, Corning Hazelton, Inc., Vienna, Va.
WILLIAM E. HALPERIN, National Institute for Occupational Safety and Health, Atlanta, Ga.
DANIEL KREWSKI, Health Canada, Ottowa, Ont.
THOMAS E. MCKONE, University of California School of Public Health, Berkeley, Calif.
MICHELE A. MEDINSKY, Chemical Industry Institute of Toxicology, Research Triangle Park, N.C.
JOHN L. O'DONOGHUE, Eastman Kodak Company, Rochester, N.Y.
ROBERT SNYDER, Environmental and Occupational Health Sciences Institute, Piscataway, N.J.
BERNARD M. WAGNER, Wagner Associates, Inc., Millburn, N.J.
ANNETTA P. WATSON, Oak Ridge National Laboratory, Oak Ridge, Tenn.
HANSPETER R. WITSCHI, University of California, Davis, Calif.
GAROLD S. YOST, University of Utah, Salt Lake City, Utah

Staff

KULBIR S. BAKSHI, Program Director for the Committee on Toxicology
SUSAN N.J. PANG, Research Associate
ABIGAIL STACK, Research Associate
RUTH E. CROSSGROVE, Publications Manager
KATHRINE IVERSON, Manager of the Toxicology Information Center
CATHERINE M. KUBIK, Senior Program Assistant
LINDA V. LEONARD, Senior Project Assistant
LUCY V. FUSCO, Project Assistant

BOARD ON ENVIRONMENTAL STUDIES AND TOXICOLOGY

GORDON ORIANS (*Chair*), University of Washington, Seattle, Wash.
DONALD MATTISON (*Vice-Chair*), University of Pittsburgh, Pittsburgh, Pa.
MAY R. BERENBAUM, University of Illinois, Urbana, Ill.
EULA BINGHAM, University of Cincinnati, Cincinnati, Ohio
PAUL BUSCH, Malcolm Pirnie, Inc., White Plains, N.Y.
GEORGE P. DASTON, The Procter & Gamble Co., Cincinnati, Ohio
PETER L. DEFUR, Virginia Commonwealth University, Richmond, Va.
DAVID L. EATON, University of Washington, Seattle, Wash.
ROBERT A. FROSCH, Harvard University, Cambridge, Mass.
MARK HARWELL, University of Miami, Miami, Fla.
BARBARA HULKA, University of North Carolina, Chapel Hill, N.C.
DANIEL KREWSKI, Health Canada and University of Ottawa, Ottawa, Ont.
RAYMOND C. LOEHR, The University of Texas, Austin, Tex.
JAMES A. MACMAHON, Utah State University, Logan, Utah
MARIO J. MOLINA, Massachusetts Institute of Technology, Cambridge, Mass.
WARREN MUIR, Hampshire Research Institute, Alexandria, Va.
GEOFFREY PLACE, Hilton Head, S.C.
MARGARET STRAND, Bayh, Connaughton and Malone, Washington, D.C.
BAILUS WALKER, JR., Howard University, Washington, D.C.
DIANA WALL, Colorado State University, Ft. Collins, Colo.
GERALD N. WOGAN, Massachusetts Institute of Technology, Cambridge, Mass.
TERRY F. YOSIE, Ruder Finn Inc., Washington, D.C.

Senior Staff

JAMES J. REISA, Director
DAVID J. POLICANSKY, Associate Director, Program Director for Applied Ecology
CAROL A. MACZKA, Program Director for Toxicology and Risk Assessment
LEE R. PAULSON, Program Director for Resource Management
RAYMOND A. WASSEL, Program Director for Environmental Sciences and Engineering
KULBIR BAKSHI, Program Director for the Committee on Toxicology

COMMISSION ON LIFE SCIENCES

THOMAS D. POLLARD *(Chair)*, The Salk Institute, La Jolla, Calif.
FREDERICK R. ANDERSON, Cadwalader, Wickersham & Taft, Washington, D.C.
JOHN C. BAILAR III, University of Chicago, Chicago, Ill.
PAUL BERG, Stanford University School of Medicine, Stanford, Calif.
JOANNA BURGER, Rutgers University, Piscataway, N.J.
SHARON L. DUNWOODY, University of Wisconsin, Madison, Wisc.
JOHN L. EMMERSON, Portland, Oreg.
NEAL L. FIRST, University of Wisconsin, Madison, Wisc.
URSULA W. GOODENOUGH, Washington University, St. Louis, Mo.
HENRY W. HEIKKINEN, University of Northern Colorado, Greeley, Colo.
HANS J. KENDE, Michigan State University, East Lansing, Mich.
CYNTHIA K. KENYON, University of California, San Francisco, Calif.
DAVID M. LIVINGSTON, Dana-Farber Cancer Institute, Boston, Mass.
THOMAS E. LOVEJOY, Smithsonian Institution, Washington, D.C.
DONALD R. MATTISON, University of Pittsburgh, Pittsburgh, Pa.
JOSEPH E. MURRAY, Wellesley Hills, Mass.
EDWARD E. PENHOET, Chiron Corporation, Emeryville, Calif.
MALCOLM C. PIKE, University of Southern California, Los Angeles, Calif.
JONATHAN M. SAMET, The Johns Hopkins University, Baltimore, Md.
CHARLES F. STEVENS, The Salk Institute, La Jolla, Calif.
JOHN L. VANDEBERG, Southwest Foundation for Biomedical Research, San Antonio, Tex.

PAUL GILMAN, Executive Director

OTHER REPORTS OF THE
BOARD ON ENVIRONMENTAL STUDIES AND TOXICOLOGY

Research Priorities for Airborne Particulate Matter: I. Immediate Priorities and a Long-Range Research Portfolio (1998)
The National Research Council's Committee on Toxicology: The First 50 Years, 1947-1997 (1998)
Carcinogens and Anticarcinogens in the Human Diet: A Comparison of Naturally Occurring Synthetic and Natural Substances (1996)
Upstream: Salmon and Society in the Pacific Northwest (1996)
Science and the Endangered Species Act (1995)
Wetlands: Characteristics and Boundaries (1995)
Biologic Markers (Urinary Toxicology (1995), Immunotoxicology (1992), Environmental Neurotoxicology (1992), Pulmonary Toxicology (1989), Reproductive Toxicology (1989))
Review of EPA's Environmental Monitoring and Assessment Program (three reports, 1994-1995)
Science and Judgment in Risk Assessment (1994)
Ranking Hazardous Sites for Remedial Action (1994)
Pesticides in the Diets of Infants and Children (1993)
Issues in Risk Assessment (1993)
Setting Priorities for Land Conservation (1993)
Protecting Visibility in National Parks and Wilderness Areas (1993)
Biologic Markers in Immunotoxicology (1992)
Dolphins and the Tuna Industry (1992)
Hazardous Materials on the Public Lands (1992)
Science and the National Parks (1992)
Animals as Sentinels of Environmental Health Hazards (1991)
Assessment of the U.S. Outer Continental Shelf Environmental Studies Program, Volumes I-IV (1991-1993)
Human Exposure Assessment for Airborne Pollutants (1991)
Monitoring Human Tissues for Toxic Substances (1991)
Rethinking the Ozone Problem in Urban and Regional Air Pollution (1991)
Decline of the Sea Turtles (1990)
Tracking Toxic Substances at Industrial Facilities (1990)

*Copies of these reports may be ordered from
the National Academy Press
(800) 624-6242 or (202) 334-3313*

OTHER REPORTS OF THE COMMITTEE ON TOXICOLOGY

Review of Acute Human-Toxicity Estimates for Selected Chemical-Warfare Agents (1997)
Toxicity of Military Smokes and Obscurants, Volume 1 (1997)
Toxicologic Assessment of the Army's Zinc Cadmium Dispersion Tests (1997)
Toxicity of Alternatives to Chlorofluorocarbons: HFC-134a and HCFC-123 (1996)
Permissible Exposure Levels for Selected Military Fuel Vapors (1996)
Spacecraft Maximum Allowable Concentrations for Selected Airborne Contaminants, Volume 1 (1994), Volume 2 (1996), and Volume 3 (1996)
Nitrate and Nitrite in Drinking Water (1995)
Guidelines for Chemical Warfare Agents in Military Field Drinking Water (1995)
Review of the U.S. Naval Medical Research Institute's Toxicology Program (1994)
Health Effects of Permethrin-Impregnated Army Battle-Dress Uniforms (1994)
Health Effects of Ingested Fluoride (1993)
Guidelines for Developing Community Emergency Exposure Levels for Hazardous Substances (1993)
Guidelines for Developing Spacecraft Maximum Allowable Concentrations for Space Station Contaminants (1992)
Review of the U.S. Army Environmental Hygiene Agency Toxicology Division (1991)
Permissible Exposure Levels and Emergency Exposure Guidance Levels for Selected Airborne Contaminants (1991)

The National Academy of Sciences is a private, nonprofit, self-perpetuating society of distinguished scholars engaged in scientific and engineering research, dedicated to the furtherance of science and technology and to their use for the general welfare. Upon the authority of the charter granted to it by the Congress in 1863, the Academy has a mandate that requires it to advise the federal government on scientific and technical matters. Dr. Bruce Alberts is president of the National Academy of Sciences.

The National Academy of Engineering was established in 1964, under the charter of the National Academy of Sciences, as a parallel organization of outstanding engineers. It is autonomous in its administration and in the selection of its members, sharing with the National Academy of Sciences the responsibility for advising the federal government. The National Academy of Engineering also sponsors engineering programs aimed at meeting national needs, encourages education and research, and recognizes the superior achievements of engineers. Dr. William A. Wulf is president of the National Academy of Engineering.

The Institute of Medicine was established in 1970 by the National Academy of Sciences to secure the services of eminent members of appropriate professions in the examination of policy matters pertaining to the health of the public. The Institute acts under the responsibility given to the National Academy of Sciences by its congressional charter to be an adviser to the federal government and, upon its own initiative, to identify issues of medical care, research, and education. Dr. Kenneth I. Shine is president of the Institute of Medicine.

The National Research Council was organized by the National Academy of Sciences in 1916 to associate the broad community of science and technology with the Academy's purposes of furthering knowledge and advising the federal government. Functioning in accordance with general policies determined by the Academy, the Council has become the principal operating agency of both the National Academy of Sciences and the National Academy of Engineering in providing services to the government, the public, and the scientific and engineering communities. The Council is administered jointly by both Academies and the Institute of Medicine. Dr. Bruce M. Alberts and Dr. William A. Wulf are chairman and vice chairman, respectively, of the National Research Council.

PREFACE

THE U.S. Air Force is developing a computer model, called the Launch Area Toxic Risk Analysis (LATRA) model, to assist commanders at Cape Canaveral and Vandenberg Air Force Base in determining when it is safe to launch rocket vehicles. LATRA estimates the incidence and types of adverse health effects that might occur in military and civilian populations exposed to the ground cloud created by rocket exhaust during a normal launch or during a catastrophic abort of a rocket that is destroyed near the ground.

This report is intended to assist the Air Force in further development of the LATRA model to ensure that the toxicity criteria used to predict health effects are scientifically valid and protective of military and civilian populations. In this report, the Subcommittee on Rocket-Emission Toxicants of the National Research Council's Committee on Toxicology evaluates the toxicity data for three rocket-emission toxicants: hydrogen chloride (HCl), nitrogen dioxide (NO_2), and nitric acid (HNO_3). The subcommittee also evaluates the exposure-response functions in the LATRA model; the functions translate exposure estimates into probabilities of health effects in populations near a launch site.

The subcommittee wishes to thank Col. Gene Killan and Mr. Tim Clapp of Peterson Air Force Base for their support of this project, and Mr. John P. Hinz and Dr. David R. Mattie of the Armstrong Laboratory at Brooks Air Force Base, Dr. Lloyd L. Philipson of ACTA Incorporated, Dr. Jeffrey I. Daniels of Lawrence Livermore National Laboratory, and Dr. Darryl Dargitz of Vandenberg Air Force Base for providing the subcommittee with information on the development and structure of the LATRA model.

Preface

This report has been reviewed by individuals chosen for their diverse perspectives and technical expertise, in accordance with procedures approved by the NRC's Report Review Committee. The purpose of this independent review is to provide candid and critical comments that will assist the NRC in making the published report as sound as possible and to ensure that the report meets institutional standards for objectivity, evidence, and responsiveness to the study charge. The content of the review comments and draft manuscript remain confidential to protect the integrity of the deliberative process. The subcommittee wishes to thank the following individuals, who are neither officials nor employees of the NRC, for their participation in the review of this report: Robert T. Drew of Hague, Va.; Yves Alarie of the University of Pittsburgh; Richard B. Schlesinger of New York University Medical Center; Matthew S. Bogdanffy of E.I. du Pont de Nemours; Sati Mazumdar of the University of Pittsburgh; and Calvin Campbell Willhite of the California Environmental Protection Agency. These reviewers have provided many constructive comments and suggestions; it must be emphasized, however, that the authoring subcommittee and the NRC are responsible for the final content of this report.

We are also grateful for the assistance of the NRC staff in the preparation of this report. In particular, the subcommittee wishes to acknowledge Carol A. Maczka, director of the Toxicology and Risk Assessment Program of the Board on Environmental Studies and Toxicology; Kulbir S. Bakshi, program director for the Committee on Toxicology; and Margaret E. McVey, staff officer for the subcommittee. Other staff members who contributed to this effort are Ruth E. Crossgrove, editor; Linda V. Leonard, senior program assistant; and Lucy Fusco, project assistant.

Finally, we would like to thank the members of the subcommittee for their valuable expertise and dedicated efforts throughout the preparation of this report.

Donald E. Gardner, Ph.D.
Chair, Subcommittee on
Rocket Emission Toxicants

Rogene F. Henderson, Ph.D.
Chair, Committee on Toxicology

CONTENTS

ABBREVIATIONS xv

EXECUTIVE SUMMARY 1

1   INTRODUCTION 10
    Development of LATRA, 11
    Organization of this Report, 12

2   DESCRIPTION OF THE LAUNCH AREA TOXIC RISK ANALYSIS
    (LATRA) MODEL 14
    Toxicity of Rocket Emissions, 15
    Identification of Sensitive Populations, 15
    Definition of Severity of Effects, 17
    Selection of the Exposure-Response Model and
       Independent Variable, 18
    Quantification of the Exposure-Response Functions, 19
    Representation of Uncertainties, 22

3   SUBPOPULATIONS SENSITIVE TO AIR CONTAMINATION 24
    Literature Review for Sensitive Subpopulations, 24
    Chemical-Specific Variation in Human Sensitivity, 26
    Limitations of Existing Studies, 29
    Common Risk-Assessment Practices for Sensitive
       Subpopulations, 31
    Defining Sensitive Populations, 32
    Conclusions and Recommendations, 33

Contents

4   EFFECT SEVERITY 37
Precedent for Severity Descriptors, 37
LATRA's Use of the Term "Severity," 41
Conclusions and Recommendations, 42

5   EVALUATION OF THE LATRA EXPOSURE-RESPONSE FUNCTIONS 45
The LATRA-ERF Model, 46
Alternative Approaches, 55
Conclusions and Recommendations, 61

6   EXPOSURE-RESPONSE FUNCTIONS FOR ROCKET-EMISSION TOXICANTS 67
Nitric Acid, 67
Hydrogen Chloride, 70
Nitrogen Dioxide, 76
Continuous (Nonquantal) Measurements, 79
Conclusions and Recommendations, 82

REFERENCES 84

APPENDIX A: AIR FORCE EXPOSURE LIMITS FOR ROCKET EMISSIONS 90

APPENDIX B: DEFINITIONS OF CURRENT EXPOSURE GUIDANCE LEVELS 98

APPENDIX C: AMERICAN THORACIC SOCIETY'S LIST OF ADVERSE RESPIRATORY HEALTH EFFECTS 103

APPENDIX D: ACUTE TOXICITY OF HYDROGEN CHLORIDE 105

APPENDIX E: ACUTE TOXICITY OF NITROGEN DIOXIDE 147

APPENDIX F: ACUTE TOXICITY OF NITRIC ACID 197

ABBREVIATIONS

ACGIH	American Conference of Governmental Industrial Hygienists
AFB	Air Force Base
ATS	American Thoracic Society
BAL	bronchoalveolar lavage;
CEL	continuous exposure limit, now called CEGL (see below)
CEGL	continuous exposure guidance level (NRC guideline)
COT	Committee on Toxicology
CT	product of exposure concentration and time
DOD	U.S. Department of Defense
DHHS	Department of Human Health Services
EEC	estimated exposure concentration
EEGL	emergency exposure guidance level (NRC guideline)
EEL	emergency exposure limit, now called EEGL (see above)
ERF	exposure-response function
EPA	U.S. Environmental Protection Agency
ERPG	Emergency Response Planning Guideline
FDA	U.S. Food and Drug Administration
GSD	geometric standard deviation
HCl	hydrogen chloride
HNO_3	nitric acid
ICBM	intercontinental ballistic missile
IDLH	immediately dangerous to life and health
LATRA	Launch Area Toxic Risk Analysis
LC_{50}	lethal concentration for 50% of the test animals
LCT_{50}	concentration multiplied by exposure time that is lethal to 50% of the test animals

ABBREVIATIONS

LD_{50}	lethal dose for 50% of the test animals
LOAEL	lowest-observed-adverse-effect level
LOC	level of concern (EPA guideline)
N_2O_4	nitrogen tetroxide
NAS	National Academy of Sciences
NHIS	National Health Interview Survey
NIOSH	National Institute for Occupational Safety and Health
NO_2	nitrogen dioxide
NOAEL	no-observed-adverse-effect level
NOEL	no-observed-effect level
NRC	National Research Council
OEL	occupational exposure limit
OSHA	Occupational Safety and Health Administration
PEL	permissible exposure level (OSHA standard)
PM-10	particulate matter less than 10 μm in diameter
PMN	polymorphonuclear neutrophils
RD_{50}	concentration (or dose) that produces a 50% decrease in respiratory rate
REEDM	Rocket Exhaust Effluent Diffusion Model
REL	recommended exposure limit (NIOSH recommendation)
REWG	Rocket Emissions Working Group
RTV	reference toxicity value
SPEGL	short-term public emergency guidance level (NRC guideline)
STEL	short-term exposure limit (NRC guideline)
STPL	short-term public limit (NRC guideline)
TLV	threshold limit value (ACGIH guideline)
TWA	time-weighted average
VAFB	Vandenberg Air Force Base

Assessment of Exposure-Response Functions for Rocket-Emission Toxicants

SUMMARY

WHEN deciding whether to launch a rocket under prevailing weather conditions, commanders at Vandenberg Air Force Base (VAFB) in California and at Cape Canaveral Air Station (CCAS) in Florida must evaluate the possibility that toxic concentrations of wind-blown rocket emissions might reach military or civilian populations. To assist commanders in estimating the risk of such exposures, the Air Force is developing the Launch Area Toxic Risk Analysis (LATRA) model. It contains two major components: (1) a dispersion model that predicts downwind exposure concentrations and (2) exposure-response functions (ERFs) that relate the estimated exposure concentrations to expected health effects.

In 1995, the Air Force Air Space Command asked the National Research Council (NRC) for an independent review of the ERFs in LATRA. The NRC was asked to focus on the toxicity of the three major rocket emissions — hydrogen chloride (HCl), nitrogen dioxide (NO_2), and nitric acid (HNO_3) — and several characteristics of LATRA ERFs, including the identification of sensitive populations; definition of severity of effects; selection of independent variables in each exposure-response model; choice of appropriate analytic form for the ERFs (e.g., lognormal or probit); quantification of ERFs for each of the emissions; and representation and propagation of uncertainties associated with the LATRA-ERF model. The NRC assigned this project to the Committee on Toxicology (COT), which convened the Subcommittee on Rocket-Emission Toxicants to respond to the request. Subcommittee members were chosen for their expertise in inhalation toxicology, pharmacology, biostatistics, risk assessment, and environmental health, and they worked without compensation in national service, as do all NRC committee members. This report presents the subcommittee's evaluations, conclusions, and recommendations.

DESCRIPTION OF THE LATRA MODEL

The LATRA model is designed to estimate the probabilities of mild and serious health effects from exposing specified human subpopulations to estimated concentrations of specific rocket emissions. For each emission, exposure-response functions (ERFs) were developed to relate estimated exposure concentrations to expected health effects. At present, separate ERFs are derived for "sensitive" and "normal" segments of the general population. An ERF is specified by two points: a lower concentration assumed to be associated with a 1% incidence of a particular effect, and an upper concentration assumed to be associated with a 99% incidence of a particular effect. An ERF is fit to the two concentration-versus-incidence points using a log-probit model (equivalent to assuming a lognormal distribution of the probability of effect). The resulting curve is then used to calculate the expected health effects and the risk profile for each population subgroup. A different procedure would be used to establish ERFs for carcinogenic emissions; however, the ERFs currently included in LATRA are not for substances known or suspected to be carcinogenic.

To set the 1% effect levels for sensitive populations, the Air Force considered the National Research Council's short-term public emergency guidance levels (SPEGLs) and other published exposure concentrations estimated to be safe for exposures of the general public. In establishing the 1% effect levels for normal populations, the Air Force considered exposure concentrations independently estimated to be safe for workers. The 99% effect levels were set 5-fold higher than the 1% effect levels for sensitive populations and 10-fold higher than the 1% effect levels for normal populations to reflect the assumed greater range in sensitivity among members of the normal population.

The subgroups considered sensitive to the rocket emissions modeled by LATRA are children (less than 15 years of age), the elderly (more than 64 years of age), and all persons with bronchitis, asthma, or other physiological stress, especially upper-respiratory ailments. The remainder of the population is considered normal.

In the LATRA model, a mild effect is defined as temporary irritation with no organic damage, and a serious (or severe) effect is defined as organic damage requiring medical treatment.

The LATRA model operates as a Monte Carlo simulation. A binomial model is used to simulate the variance (uncertainty) associated with the predicted number of people affected. The potential for combined effects of exposure to more than one compound is estimated by developing joint probabilities of effect from the individual toxicants' probabilities of effect. The LATRA model estimates of the total number of people at risk of health effects from a launch are based on (1) the risks associated with a normal launch, (2) the probability of a normal launch, (3) the risks associated with a catastrophic abort, and (4) the probability of a catastrophic abort.

THE SUBCOMMITTEE'S CONCLUSIONS AND RECOMMENDATIONS

In general, the subcommittee found the basic premise of the LATRA model—using exposure-versus-incidence-of-response models to predict the incidence of effects in humans—to be reasonable, but the available toxicological data on the specified rocket-emission toxicants are currently insufficient to support the ERFs used in the LATRA model. The subcommittee's specific conclusions and recommendations with respect to the toxicological components of LATRA, and possible alternative approaches recommended by the subcommittee, are described below.

TOXICOLOGICAL DATA BASE

The toxicity data available for HCl, NO_2, and HNO_3 are sufficient to identify no-observed-effect levels (NOELs) for humans and to indicate varying differences in sensitivity at low exposure concentrations between individuals with asthma and healthy individuals. The available data also are sufficient to estimate thresholds for mild, moderate, and severe effects for HCl and NO_2, but not for HNO_3. However, the only exposure-response data useful for predicting the proportion of individuals that might be affected by exposure to those compounds appear to be the data on mortality and severe effects in animals exposed to HCl and the data on mortality in animals exposed to NO_2. Thus, the subcommittee found that the toxicity data on HCl, NO_2, and HNO_3 are insufficient to support the development of separate ERFs for mild and serious effects in sensitive and normal human populations.

IDENTIFICATION OF SENSITIVE SUBGROUPS

The subcommittee recognizes that interindividual differences in toxicological responses to chemical exposure are a major area of public-health concern. The causes of these differences include age, sex, genetic background, nutritional status, pre-existing diseases, and life style. The subcommittee does not believe that age (e.g., individuals over 64 years of age) should be the principal attribute to identify a segment of the sensitive population. The subcommittee believes that a more accurate assessment of the number of potentially sensitive individuals in the population near the launch sites can be obtained by basing sensitivity on the estimated prevalence of health conditions likely to render a person sensitive rather than by basing sensitivity on indirect measurements such as age. For adults, information on the age-specific incidence of diseases likely to increase individuals' sensitivity to rocket-emission toxicants can be used with information on the ages of the exposed individuals. Although sensitivity within the adult subpopulation might be due to the presence of certain diseases rather than to age, children might indeed be a potentially susceptible population, even when healthy. That potential could be due to such factors as differences in ventilation rate in children compared with healthy adults. The National Health Interview Survey (NHIS), available from the U.S. Bureau of Census, could be used to obtain information on age-specific disease incidence. The subcommittee recognizes that children might represent a potential susceptible population, even when healthy.

The LATRA model includes separate ERFs for sensitive and normal populations. The subcommittee endorses explicit consideration of potentially sensitive subgroups; however, as mentioned above, it found the toxicity data available for the rocket-emission toxicants inadequate to define separate ERFs for the two subgroups. Available data support only the derivation of different thresholds of effect in sensitive and normal individuals. The toxicity information available for the three rocket emissions indicates that for short-duration exposures (i.e., 1 hr or less), sensitive individuals begin to respond at lower concentrations than normal individuals by a factor of 10 for NO_2, a factor of 3 for HCl, and a factor of 20 for HNO_3.

DEFINITION OF SEVERITY OF EFFECTS

The Air Force asked the subcommittee to consider how best to define three categories of severity of effects: mild, moderate, and serious. The subcommittee believes that categorizing specific effects into such severity categories is an acceptable approach. The subcommittee defined mild, moderate, and serious effects as follows. Mild effects are reversible within 48 hr and do not interfere with normal activity or require medical attention. Moderate effects are irreversible effects that do not alter organ function or interfere with normal activity, or they are reversible effects that alter organ function or interfere with normal activity. Persons experiencing moderate effects might seek medical attention. Severe effects are irreversible effects that alter organ function or interfere with normal activities. Severe effects usually require medical attention. Those definitions are specific for exposures to rocket emissions and might not be applicable to other exposure scenarios or toxicants.

STRUCTURE OF THE LATRA-ERF MODEL

In principle, the LATRA-ERF model is a valid concept, but the subcommittee does not endorse use of the LATRA-ERF model as it is currently constructed. The ERFs give the appearance of substantial accuracy; yet, they are not adequately supported by toxicological information. Consequently, a user of the LATRA-ERF model might believe that the model is more reliable than it actually is for estimating risk. In the interim, the subcommittee instead recommends that the hazard-quotient approach be used to characterize risks for sensitive and normal populations, as described below. However, if the Air Force wants to pursue the LATRA-ERF model, there are ways to improve components of the model, as described below.

The ERFs in the LATRA model are currently based on 1-hr time-weighted-average concentrations and ceiling values. The subcommittee believes that 1 hr is too long because of the typical speed with which the ground cloud of emissions from a rocket launch passes over a given exposure location; increments of 10 to 30 min would be more representative of the exposure situation, covering the total duration of exposure. The LATRA model is capable of incrementing exposures. The subcommittee endorses the use of ceiling values for noncumulative effects. It also identified certain effects for which the product of exposure concentration and time (C × T) would be appropriate: for example, severe effects and mortality for HCl and NO_2. For effects for which the relationship between effect and the product of C × T is unknown, the subcommittee recommends that sensitivity studies be conducted to determine how the selection of the independent variables for the ERF influences the LATRA model's output. If time-weighted-average concentrations for 10 and 30 min are used, for example, those results should be compared with the results of using C × T as the independent variable.

A weakness of the current derivation of LATRA ERFs is that the dose-response model for predicting incidence (a log-probit model) is based on health-protective or "safe" levels that have no specified relation to the incidence of effects. The subcommittee does not believe that it is appropriate to interpret a safe level as a 1% incidence level for mild effects. The true incidence could be higher but is likely to be lower and presumably near or at zero. An accurate ERF could be used to predict the incidence below the 1% level. The subcommittee also does not believe that it is necessarily appropriate, in the absence of supporting data, to interpret a concentration that is 5- or 10-fold higher than that causing a 1% incidence level as the concentration at which all individuals are likely to show effects. That level provides a relatively steep ERF that might be conservative above a 1% incidence level, but might not be appropriate for the more likely scenario of exposure below a 1% incidence level. Combining the 1% and 99% incidence-versus-exposure values to construct a model for predicting the incidence is a judgmental process that lacks any direct measurements from either epidemiological or toxicological data.

To the extent possible, the Air Force should use end-point-specific incidence data to develop end-point-specific ERFs. However, with the exception of mortality and a few other end points, incidence data for HCl, NO_2, and HNO_3 are not available. Without incidence data on humans or animals, it is difficult to endorse exposure-response models that predict incidence. Until end-point-specific data become available for

HCl, NO_2, and HNO_3, the Air Force could attempt to validate the model against other compounds, such as chlorine gas and ammonia, that are likely to have adequate data on humans.

The subcommittee recommends that the Air Force generate appropriate toxicity data to calibrate and validate the proposed model. The investments in appropriate testing procedures, at this time, would be worth the effort by improving the model's predictibility and reducing the uncertainty. Such studies should, at a minimum, examine concentration times, time responses, and include adequate histopathology. Appropriate toxicity data will allow the Air Force to calibrate its model on the basis of sound data.

Until more data become available or an expert-elicitation process can be carried out to estimate incidence for end points with no incidence data, the subcommittee believes that a hazard-quotient model would be more appropriate. For the hazard-quotient model, estimates of the number of people at risk would be based on the number of people with exposures above a reference exposure level that is unlikely to cause adverse health effects. The ratio of the exposure concentrations to reference exposure levels might also be useful. The hazard-quotient model could be used to estimate how many people might be at risk of moderate or severe effects if the Air Force is willing to accept the level of uncertainty associated with exposure values identified as a threshold exposure for moderate and severe effects.

Under the LATRA model, separate ERFs are developed for sensitive and normal populations. However, a properly constructed probit model can portray a wide variation in human sensitivity within a single exposure-response function. Moreover, available data are insufficient to quantify different ERFs for sensitive and normal populations. Thus, the subcommittee cannot support the use of specific ERFs for sensitive and normal populations, although it does support the use of different thresholds for effect if the hazard-quotient approach is used to characterize risk.

In the absence of incidence data to construct ERFs for sensitive subgroups, the hazard-quotient approach could be used to characterize risk. When deriving a hazard quotient, the common practice is to use animal or human data to define a low- or no-effect level. That level is then divided by an appropriate uncertainty factor to yield an allowable exposure level. The hazard quotient is the ratio of an observed or predicted exposure to an allowable exposure. The allowable exposure level would be set at a lower value by selecting an uncertainty factor that is sufficient to protect sensitive individuals.

To avoid embedding value judgments in the scientific exposure-response analysis, ERFs should be developed first by health end point. After considering all the end points, decisions can then be made on which exposure concentrations to associate with mild, moderate, and severe effects. Incidence dose-response data are lacking for all but severe end points for HCl and NO_2 and are altogether lacking for HNO_3. It is possible, however, to estimate a reference exposure that is unlikely to cause mild effects for all three of the rocket emissions. In addition, reference exposures for moderate and severe effects can be estimated for HCl and NO_2 (see Appendices D and E), although there are large uncertainties concerning the time-dependence of those estimates. Those reference exposures could be used with the hazard-quotient model. The subcommittee suggests that the Air Force be especially aware to avoid making certain value judgments based on an incomplete or limited data base. Such limitations make it difficult to evaluate or predict accurately the degree to which a specific human subpopulation might be more sensitive to air contaminants than others.

The subcommittee does not recommend using the binomial model in LATRA to address uncertainty. The binomial model generates a variance that underestimates the variance associated with fitting the ERF to response data.

If an adequate data base becomes available to support the development of ERFs, sensitivity analyses should be conducted to investigate the assumptions and procedures used to construct the ERFs.

The subcommittee recommends that the Air Force evaluate potential health effects resulting from simultaneous exposure to more than one toxic rocket emission, assuming the potential for additive effects. That could be accomplished by using the hazard-index approach (i.e., adding the hazard quotients for individual chemicals) to characterize risk.

Given the complex nature and extent and pattern of injury in the respiratory tract from exposure to airborne chemicals, it is important to understand interspecies differences in their response to inhaled substances. The ability to make interspecies dosimetric comparisons is critically important for judging the applicability of various toxicological results to human exposure conditions. Selected dosimetric experiments involving laboratory animals and humans can provide valuable data on the variability in uptake according to species and the specific region within the respiratory tract where the chemical might target. New experimental dosimetric approaches, such as those involving isotope ratio mass spectroscopy and cyclotron generation of gases, offer promise for improving the ability to make scientifically defensible predictions. The subcommittee recommends that the Air Force consider including interspecies dosimetric correction factors when applicable.

Instead of presenting one risk estimate for a launch that combines the risks of a normal launch and a catastrophic abort, the subcommittee believes that it would be more appropriate for the Air Force to present separate risks for normal and aborted launches or to provide separate conditional risks and combined risks.

The Air Force should ensure that any time-weighted-average exposure estimate used to determine risk is the maximum value possible. For example, the maximum 30-min time-weighted-average concentration passing over an exposure location should be compared with a 30-min ERF or a reference exposure unlikely to cause an adverse health effect.

The subcommittee also recommends that the Air Force evaluate the relative accuracies of the exposure estimates from the rocket-exhaust dispersion model and the estimates of incidence of effects from the ERFs (or reference exposures as suggested here). If the Air Force can determine whether the exposure component or the effects component of the LATRA model is the more serious limit to the model's accuracy in predicting risk, it can invest effort in improving the less accurate component.

In summary, the LATRA-ERF model is a valid concept, but the current lack of toxicological data makes its implementation problematic. Some specific deficiencies have been noted above by the subcommittee, and some improvements in the LATRA-ERF model might be possible. In the interim, the subcommittee suggests that a hazard-quotient–hazard-index approach be considered as a possible alternative. This approach would allow an estimate of the number of people exceeding a reference exposure level below which health effects are unlikely to occur. This approach would not attempt to estimate the incidence of health effects in an exposed population.

1

INTRODUCTION

THE Air Force has developed a probabilistic health-risk model, the Launch Area Toxic Risk Analysis (LATRA) model, to assist commanders in determining the risks to military personnel and civilians from exposure to emissions from normal and failed missile and space rocket launches. The model estimates the mean number of persons who might experience mild or serious health effects and the probability of exceeding each possible number of affected individuals. The Air Force Space Command requested that the National Research Council (NRC) independently review the toxicological components of LATRA to ensure their appropriateness. Specifically, the NRC was asked to focus on the toxicity of the three major rocket emissions — hydrogen chloride (HCl), nitrogen dioxide (NO_2), and nitric acid (HNO_3) — and several characteristics of the exposure-response components of LATRA, including identification of sensitive populations; definition of mild, moderate, and severe health effects; selection of independent variable in the exposure-response model; choice of analytic form for the exposure-response model (e.g., lognormal or probit) for each of the emissions; quantification of exposure-response model for each of the emissions; and representation and propagation of the uncertainties associated with the models. The NRC assigned this project to the Committee on Toxicology (COT), which convened the Subcommittee on Rocket-Emission Toxicants to respond to the request. Subcommittee members were chosen because of their expertise in inhalation toxicology, pharmacology, biostatistics, risk assessment, and environmental health. This report presents the subcommittee's evaluations, conclusions, and recommendations.

INTRODUCTION

The remainder of this chapter provides a brief background of the development of LATRA and describes the organization of this report.

DEVELOPMENT OF LATRA

To assist commanders in making decisions on whether to launch a rocket given the weather conditions at the time of launch, the Air Force developed an atmospheric dispersion computer model, the Rocket Exhaust Effluent Diffusion Model (REEDM), which simulates the dispersion of a rocket's emissions under prevailing weather conditions. Specifically, REEDM predicts an isopleth, or "footprint," of the concentrations of specific emissions at ground level downwind of the specific launch site.

Initially, the Air Force compared the exposure concentrations predicted by REEDM for each of the emissions with acceptable human exposure levels, called tier limits. Three different tier limits were developed for military and civilian base personnel and for the communities located around the launch centers. The derivation of those tier limits is described in more detail in Appendix A. If REEDM predicted that specific populations would be exposed at concentrations higher than the appropriate tier limits, the commander would be advised to hold the launch. The Air Force later decided that acceptable human exposure levels should not exceed one tenth of the National Institute for Occupational Safety and Health (NIOSH) immediately dangerous to life and health (IDLH) levels, for occupational exposures on base, and short-term public emergency guidance levels (SPEGLs) developed by the NRC, at the breathing zone for the public (U.S. Air Force 1994). (See Appendix B for definitions of IDLH and SPEGL values.)

That policy remained in effect until November of 1994, when a Peacekeeper launch was delayed several times, and then postponed, because REEDM predicted, based on forecasted lift-off weather conditions, that a nearby town would be exposed to HCl at concentrations that would exceed the SPEGL. That cancellation cost the Air Force hundreds of thousands of dollars. The Air Force subsequently estimated that the use of the 1-hr SPEGL of 1 ppm as a maximum allowable concentration (i.e., a ceiling limit value) for HCl reduced the probability of a rocket being launched as scheduled from nearly 100% (prior to 1994) to about 27%, substantially increasing the overall costs of rocket launches. That information resulted in a reevaluation of the HCl toxicity criteria and increased emphasis on implementing a probabilistic model, LATRA, to replace the simple comparison of acceptable human exposure levels with REEDM isopleths.

The LATRA model is designed to estimate the probabilities of various adverse health effects from exposing specified human populations to specific toxic emissions during rocket launches. It includes two major components: (1) a version of REEDM to predict downwind exposure concentrations and (2) exposure-response functions (ERFs) that relate the estimated exposure concentrations to expected health effects. LATRA estimates the mean number of people affected and the complete risk profile (the curve of the probability of exceeding each possible number of individuals affected) resulting from the rocket emissions from normal and failed rocket launches.

ORGANIZATION OF THIS REPORT

The remainder of this report is organized in six chapters with accompanying appendices. Chapter 2 describes the LATRA model and issues concerning its exposure-response components in more detail. Additional information on the rocket emissions, the derivation of the Air Force tier limits, and the relationship of those limits to the toxicity values used to develop LATRA are described in Appendix A. Definitions of established toxicity reference values that the Air Force considered in developing LATRA are provided in Appendix B. Chapter 3 provides the subcommittee's evaluation, conclusions, and recommendations concerning the identification of sensitive populations in light of the data available for the three rocket-emission toxicants and similar compounds. Chapter 4 provides the subcommittee's evaluation, conclusions, and recommendations concerning the definition of severity of effects. (Appendix C provides supplementary information for Chapter 4). Chapter 5 provides the subcommittee's evaluation of the structure of the LATRA-ERF model with respect to the characteristics the Air Force identified for review (noted above) and identifies possible alternative approaches to establishing exposure-response relationships or estimating incidence of effects. Chapter 5 concludes with suggestions for improving the LATRA-ERF model and for alternative approaches to estimating health risks for rocket emissions. Chapter 6 provides examples of implementing the suggested alternative approaches for developing ERFs for HCl, NO_2, and HNO_3 on the basis of the available exposure-response data for those compounds, which are presented in Appendices D, E, and F, respectively.

2

DESCRIPTION OF THE LAUNCH AREA TOXIC RISK ANALYSIS (LATRA) MODEL

As noted in Chapter 1, the LATRA model is used to define human-health risks associated with rocket-launch scenarios (i.e., normal launches with different rocket-fuel types and accident scenarios). Coupling source characteristics of the toxic agents under consideration—HCl, NO_2, and HNO_3—with real-time meteorological data, a dispersion model (REEDM) is used to simulate exposures (i.e., to predict concentration-time profiles at receptor locations). The exposure-response functions (ERFs) in LATRA translate exposure estimates from REEDM into probabilities of health effects in specified severity categories in the human population. At present, separate ERFs are developed for two segments of the population: "sensitive" and "normal" populations. Within each segment, the model incorporates separate ERFs for "mild" and "serious" health effects. The ERFs included in LATRA at present are lognormal for noncarcinogenic substances and linear, passing through the origin, for carcinogenic substances. When sufficient data are available to support a nonlinear ERF for a carcinogen, the Air Force should consider modeling such data.

At each receptor location modeled by REEDM, the ERFs are applied to the number of individuals estimated from census data to be present in both population subgroups at that location. For each severity category, the ERF is the probability, P_E, per individual of an effect, Y, exceeding a given severity category, S (mild or serious) given an exposure concentration and duration. That is,

DESCRIPTION OF THE LATRA MODEL

$$P_E(S,C,T) = P(Y \geq S/C,T),$$

where $P_E(S,C,T)$ is the ERF for an exposure characterized by concentration, C, and time or duration of exposure, T, and is equal to the probability of the severity equaling or exceeding a given severity category, S, at a specified exposure concentration, C, and duration, T.

As indicated in Chapter 1, the task of the subcommittee was to review and provide recommendations on several issues surrounding the exposure-response components of the LATRA model. Further description of the model and issues surrounding those components is provided below.

TOXICITY OF ROCKET EMISSIONS

The toxicity reference values originally used by the Air Force in the LATRA-ERF model to represent a 1%-effect level for HCl, NO_2, and HNO_3, had been established by other groups almost a decade earlier (e.g., NRC 1987, 1991). The toxicity data for those substances needed to be re-evaluated with respect to sensitive populations, severity of effect, and the availability of dose-response information. Those reevaluations are presented in Appendices D, E, and F, respectively. Use of that information to derive ERFs for LATRA is explored in Chapter 6.

IDENTIFICATION OF SENSITIVE POPULATIONS

The LATRA-ERF model divides potentially exposed populations into at least two population subgroups, sensitive and normal, and develops separate ERFs for each subgroup. Sensitive populations are defined as children (less than 15 years of age), the elderly (more than 64 years of age), and all persons with bronchitis, asthma, or other physiological stress, especially upper-respiratory ailments (Gene Killan, U.S. Air Force Space Command, personal commun., May 6, 1996). Under LATRA, the remainder of the population is considered "normal" and is assumed to be composed of healthy adults. Census data are used to determine the locations of the sensitive subgroups around a launch site (e.g., in nursing homes and schools). Because the ERFs for sensitive individuals are applied only to such locations identified by census data and only to the proportion of the population considered sensitive at these sites, they do not not protect sensitive individuals within the larger community. Sensitive subgroups are assumed to respond to the rocket-emission toxicants at lower concentrations than the normal population and to exhibit less variation in response, showing a steeper increase in incidence of response with increasing exposure concentration than does the normal population. How the ERFs are actually quantified for LATRA is discussed later in this chapter in the section Quantification of the Exposure-Response Functions.

Although this approach requires quantifying separate ERFs for each population subgroup, the Air Force pointed out that it allows them to apply the ERF for healthy adults to all locations where sensitive subgroups are not found. The more conservative ERFs for sensitive individuals need be applied only to those locations where the census data indicate that there are sensitive subgroups and only to the proportion of the population considered sensitive at those locations.

Based on information supplied to the subcommittee, it appears that the Air Force adopted the elderly age cutoff of more than 64 years from an EPA definition that was used by CDC (1993) investigators when estimating populations at risk in communities that have not attained one or more National Ambient Air Quality Standards in the United States (Poitrast 1993).

The subcommittee considered several questions when evaluating the sensitivity component of the LATRA-ERF model: What characteristics are likely to make an individual more sensitive to the specific rocket-emission toxicants? What is the magnitude of the difference in sensitivity between the more-sensitive members and the more-average members of the population? Is the difference in sensitivity between those groups reflected in the concentration representing a threshold for response, the severity of response for a given concentration, the variability in response, or some combination of those attributes? What considerations for hypersensitive individuals might be appropriate? The subcommittee's evaluation, conclusions, and recommendations regarding these questions are provided in Chapter 3.

DEFINITION OF SEVERITY OF EFFECTS

The LATRA model has three health-effect severity levels, as listed below:

Mild: no damage to body organs; temporary irritation.
Significant (or severe or serious): damage to body organs; treatment required.
Fatal (considered unacceptable) (Philipson et al. 1996).

The LATRA considers two categories of severity—mild and worse and serious and worse—with separate ERFs for each.

The Air Force asked an inter-agency advisory panel, the Rocket Emissions Working Group (REWG) (see Appendix A), to identify what signs or symptoms would be expected to accompany mild and severe effects. For an acute (minutes to 1 hr) exposure to irritant gases that are relatively soluble in aqueous solution (e.g., HCl), REWG identified a mild response to be a transient irritation of the eyes, skin, and upper airways (nasopharyngeal and upper tracheobronchial tree) (Gene Killan, U.S. Air Force Space Command, personal commun., May 6, 1996). REWG identified likely responses as sneezing, nasal catarrh (i.e., inflammation of mucous membrane), unpleasant smell or taste, throat soreness, smarting of the eyes, and lacrimation (tearing). REWG identified a severe response to be a reversible or irreversible response that might require medical intervention, especially when the central airways of the tracheobronchial tree are involved. REWG identified signs and symptoms of severe effects as coughing, sputum, pain, chest constriction, bronchospasm, shortness of breath, and wheezing.

The subcommittee evaluated the approach of categorizing health effects by severity and of developing separate ERFs for each severity category. Also, because the Air Force stated that a category reflecting moderate effects would assist in making launch decisions, the subcommittee evaluated how to define three levels of effect severity—mild, moderate, and severe—in a way that is both scientifically sound and meaningful to an Air Force commander. The subcommittee's evaluation, conclusions, and recommendations concerning the approach and definition of severity categories are presented in Chapter 4.

SELECTION OF THE EXPOSURE-RESPONSE MODEL AND INDEPENDENT VARIABLE

The ERFs included in LATRA at present are lognormal for noncarcinogenic substances and linear, passing through the origin, for carcinogenic substances. (Note: ERFs have not been developed for any carcinogenic substances to date (Philipson 1996)). ERFs for noncarcinogenic substances are actually represented by a *log-probit* model applied to either the *maximum 1-hr time-weighted-average (TWA) concentration* (C_{max}, 1-hr) or to the *ceiling concentration* (C_{max}). Because the log-probit model is equivalent to a cumulative lognormal distribution function, the LATRA ERF can be characterized generically as a model for predicting

$$P_E(S,C,T) = P(Y \geq S/C,T) = \text{lognormal}_{cml}[C_{max},1\text{-hr},\mu_1(S),s_1(S)],$$

where $\text{lognormal}_{cml}[C_{max},1\text{-hr},\mu_1(S),s_1(S)]$ is the cumulative lognormal distribution function with mean natural logarithm of concentration, $\ln(C)$, equal to $\mu_1(S)$ and standard deviation in $\ln(C)$ equal to $s_1(S)$. When a ceiling concentration is used instead of the 1-hr TWA, then the term "C_{max},1-hr" is replaced by "C_{max}," representing the ceiling concentration.

This distribution expresses the probability that a randomly selected individual within a population experiences an effect of at least severity S when the distribution of likelihood of response in that population is such that half the population will experience an effect at

$$C_{max},1\text{-hr} = \exp(\mu_1(S)),$$

and where the geometric standard deviation (GSD) of this distribution of effects of severity S is given by

$$GSD(S) = \exp(s_1(S)).$$

The GSD expresses the implicit variation in the probability of response per individual based on the assumed set points for concentrations corresponding to the 1% and 99% incidence rates.

The log probit has a sigmoidal shape. Special graph paper can be used that converts incidence (proportions or percentages) to probits so that a straight line plot of probits versus log dose is obtained. The slope

DESCRIPTION OF THE LATRA MODEL

of that line is the reciprocal of the geometric standard deviation. Specific examples are illustrated in Chapter 6.

Separate ERFs are used for the 1-hr TWA and the ceiling values; the higher probability of effect from the two curves is then used in computing the number of people likely to be affected. The REEDM dispersion model contained within LATRA does not reliably predict instantaneous peak concentrations, however. Averaging times of at least 30 min are considered the most meaningful model output (Stokes 1994), although the model does analyze exposures down to 5-min increments. The documentation supplied to the subcommittee did not specify, however, how maximum peak or TWA exposure concentrations are derived from the REEDM output for comparison with the toxicity values.

The subcommittee considered whether the two different independent variables included in LATRA—a 1-hr TWA value and a ceiling value—are the most appropriate, given what is known about the rocket-emission toxicants and given the likely duration and frequency of exposure. The subcommittee also considered what type of exposure-response model would be most appropriate for the ERFs for the three rocket-emission toxicants under evaluation and for the types of risks that LATRA is attempting to estimate. The subcommittee's evaluation, conclusions, and recommendations regarding those issues are provided in Chapter 5.

QUANTIFICATION OF THE EXPOSURE-RESPONSE FUNCTIONS

The lognormal ERFs for noncarcinogenic rocket emissions are specified at present by two symmetric percentiles: the 1 and 99 percentiles. Specifically, the values $\mu_1(S)$ and $s_1(S)$ associated with the GSD are determined by assigning to the 1% effect level of the distribution a *safe* exposure concentration and by assigning to the 99% effect level an assumed ED_{100} value (dose assumed to cause an effect in 100% of the population). Thus,

$$P_E(S,C,T) = P_E(S,C_{01},\text{1-hr}) = \text{lognormal}_{\text{cml}}[C_{\max} = C_{01}, \text{1-hr}, \mu_1(S), s_1(S)],$$

where

C_{01},1-hr = 1-hr SPEGL or other measure of safe dose,

$P_E(S,C,T) = P_E(S,C_{99},1\text{-hr}) = \text{lognormal}_{cml}[C_{max} = C_{99},1\text{-hr},\mu_1(S),s_1(S)]$,

and C_{99},1-hr = 1-hr ED_{100}.

Under those constraints,

$\mu_1(S) = (C_{01} \times C_{99})^{1/2}$, and

$s_1(S) = [\ln(C_{01}) - \ln(C_{99})]/(2 \times 2.33)$.

The lognormal curves are cut off to zero below the 1 percentile to reflect a threshold for noncancer effects and raised to 1.0 above the 99 percentile to be conservative. The assumption is that the 1% effect level represents exposures below which "essentially no one" would experience each specified severity of effect. The 99% effect level represents exposures above which "essentially everyone" would experience the specified severity of effect (Philipson 1996).

The Air Force considered SPEGLs and other established exposure concentrations considered safe for the general public when setting the 1% effect levels for sensitive populations. Similarly, the Air Force considered established exposure concentrations considered safe for workers in setting the 1% effect levels for normal populations. The 99% effect levels were set 5-fold higher than the 1% effect levels for sensitive populations and 10-fold higher than the 1% effect levels for normal populations (Philipson 1996). The documentation provided to the subcommittee did not explain the rationale for those values; however, L. Philipson (ACTA Inc., personal commun., Jan. 15-16, 1997) indicated to the subcommittee that the range of variability in response among individuals in a normal subgroup was assumed to be twice the range of variability among individuals in a sensitive subgroup. There also was consideration of NIOSH (1994) immediately dangerous to life and health (IDLH) values in developing the tier limits considered dangerous and consideration of the tier limits in identifying appropriate toxicity values for the 99% incidence values (see Chapter 1 and Appendix A). Table 2-1 lists the exposure concentrations associated with the 1% and 99% incidence values for sensitive and normal populations and mild and serious effects for the three rocket-emission toxicants.

TABLE 2-1 Exposure Concentrations Associated with the 1% and 99% Effect Levels in the LATRA-ERFs

Population	Effect Level		HCl, ppm		NO$_2$, ppm		HNO$_3$, ppm	
			1%	99%[a]	1%	99%[a]	1%	99%[a]
Sensitive	Mild		2, TWA[b,c]	10, TWA	0.2, TWA[b,c]	1.0 TWA	—	—
			10, ceiling[c]	50, ceiling	2, ceiling[c]	10, ceiling	0.3, ceiling[c]	1.5, ceiling
	Serious		—	—	2, TWA[e]	10, TWA	2.5, ceiling[e]	12.5, TWA
			20, ceiling[d]	100, ceiling	4, ceiling[e]	20, ceiling	4, ceiling[e]	20, ceiling
Normal	Mild		—	—	2, TWA[e]	20, TWA	2.5, TWA[e]	25, TWA
			10, ceiling[f]	100, ceiling	4, ceiling[e]	40, ceiling	4, ceiling[e]	40, ceiling
	Serious		—	—	4, TWA[h]	40, TWA	5, TWA[h]	50, TWA
			50, ceiling[g]	500, ceiling	8, ceiling[h]	80, ceiling	8, ceiling[h]	80, ceiling

[a]Ninety-nine percentiles are estimated as 5 times the 1 percentiles for sensitive populations (so that medians (50% response) are the square root of 5 multiplied by the 1 percentiles), 10 times the 1 percentiles for normal populations, reflecting an assumed greater variability in the normal populations and maintaining greater conservatism in the ERFs for the sensitive populations. (An ERF rises faster (has a steeper dose-response curve) when the upper limit is closer to the lower limit.)

[b]All time-weighted-average (TWA) values are for 1 hr of exposure.

[c]Interim guidance for tier 1 (general public), stated to apply to mild effect in sensitive individuals (all general public).

[d]Assumed to be 2 times the sensitive-mild-effect ceiling limit; it is believed to be conservative. (In the initial estimates, a factor of 3.5 is applied.)

[e]Previously understood tier 2 limit (see Appendix A) as mild effects in normal individuals; assumed also for serious effect in sensitive individuals.

[f]The tier 2 limit (see Appendix A) was assumed to apply here.

[g]This was understood previously to be the tier 3 limit (see Appendix A), one-half the value considered by NIOSH to be immediately dangerous to life and health (IDLH), adopted here for serious effects in normal individuals.

[h]Two times the 1 percentile for serious effects in sensitive individuals.

The subcommittee evaluated the appropriateness of this approach to quantifying the chemical-specific ERFs, including the appropriateness of using "safe" levels to represent the 1% effect level, the approach for identifying a 99% effect level, and the assumed difference in slope of the log-probit function between sensitive and normal populations. The subcommittee also considered alternative analytic models to the log-probit model and what types of chemical-specific information or data are most appropriate to use for each approach. Those evaluations, and the subcommittee's conclusions and recommendations, are also presented in Chapter 5.

REPRESENTATION OF UNCERTAINTIES

The ERFs represent a deterministic relationship between exposure concentration and the proportion of an exposed population that would exhibit an effect at a specified severity level. At each receptor location where a concentration for each rocket-emission is estimated, the number of people affected in the population at that location is calculated from the probability P_E using a binomial distribution. That is, the number of individuals in each subgroup who suffer at least an effect of severity S at the given receptor location is estimated as

$$n(N,S,C,T) = \text{sum}(i = 1, 2, \ldots N)\{i \times P_{bnml}[i,N,P_E(S,C,T)]\},$$

where n is the expected number of individuals with effects of at least severity S in a population of size N, exposed to concentration C for duration T, and P_{bnml} is the binomial distribution function that expresses the probability of observing i effects in a population of size N, when the probability of effect per individual is $P_E(S,C,T)$. In the current LATRA model, all of those binomial distributions are combined by adding their means and variances to obtain the mean and variance of the total number of people suffering effects of a given severity at all receptor locations. To derive a complete risk profile, the binomials are usually approximated by Poissons to obtain a total Poisson distribution for all possible numbers of affected individuals.

LATRA estimates the total number of people at risk from the launch on the basis of: (1) the risks associated with a normal launch, (2) the probability of a normal launch, (3) the risks associated with a catastrophic abort, and (4) the probability of a catastrophic abort. Depending on the toxicity criteria used, as well as the quantity of propellants onboard, meteorological conditions, proximity of population centers, and so forth, far greater health risks generally are expected for catastrophic aborts than for normal launches. As a consequence, the total risk estimate produced by LATRA generally reflects the risks estimated for a catastrophic abort because the risks estimated for a normal launch usually are much lower.

The potential for combined effects of exposure to more than one compound at the same time is estimated after the risk profiles for individual compounds are estimated by "developing joint probabilities of effect from the individual toxics' probabilities of effect (assuming their independence)" (Philipson et al. 1996). This assumption was considered conservative because of the high level of correlation expected among exposures to the individual toxic emissions. The mode of action of the various toxicants needs to be considered. Such an investigation might provide support for response additivity or dose additivity of the constituents in a mixture.

The subcommittee considered the relative importance of the various uncertainties associated with the LATRA-ERF model, evaluating how well the important uncertainties are represented in the model and how they should be used to qualify the risk estimates. Those evaluations and the subcommittee's conclusions and recommendations also are provided in Chapter 5.

3

SUBPOPULATIONS SENSITIVE TO AIR CONTAMINATION

THIS chapter presents the subcommittee's evaluation of the Air Force's definition of sensitive subpopulations. The subcommittee investigated whether some population subgroups are likely to be more sensitive to the rocket-emission toxicants than the general population and, if some are, (1) how much more sensitive they are and (2) how they can be identified.

This chapter is divided into six sections. The first section presents the subcommittee's evaluation of the literature reviews on populations sensitive to air pollutants published in recent years. In the second section, the subcommittee reviews the available qualitative and quantitative data on the variation in human sensitivity to specific air pollutants, including the three major rocket-emission toxicants discussed in this report. In the third section, the subcommittee identifies several limitations of those studies for purposes of risk assessment. In the fourth section, the subcommittee describes common practices for accounting for sensitive subpopulations in human health risk assessments when data on sensitivity are lacking. In the fifth section, the subcommittee evaluates the Air Force criteria for defining sensitive subpopulations. In the sixth section, the subcommittee presents its conclusions and recommendations.

LITERATURE REVIEW FOR SENSITIVE SUBPOPULATIONS

The subcommittee consulted several recent reviews focusing on variations in individual susceptibility (i.e., sensitivity) to pollutants (Brain et al. 1988; WHO 1992; NRC 1993; ATS 1996a,b).

The NRC (1993) report concluded that profound differences exist between children and adults. Because infants and children are growing and developing, they are different from adults in composition and in certain metabolic, physiological, and biochemical processes. Before full maturation, damage to a specific organ or organ system might permanently prevent normal physical maturation and increase the incidence of a variety of diseases. That possibility has been demonstrated in studies showing children's sensitivity to the irreversible effects of lead and mercury (Calabrese 1986; Klaassen et al. 1996), enhanced susceptibility to certain radiation-induced cancers (Calabrese 1978), and enhanced risk from a number of carcinogens, e.g., vinyl chloride-induced angiosarcoma (Drew et al. 1983; Calabrese 1986). In addition, certain populations of children might be more sensitive than other children to the effects of chemical agents because of physiological and biochemical factors, such as genetic predisposition, general health status, low socioeconomic status, and possible interactions with certain medications. For certain types of toxicity, children might be more resistant to certain chemical agents, and in such cases, adults might be at greater risk.

Brain et al. (1988) provided a comprehensive analysis of the general principles for variations in human sensitivity to inhaled air pollutants. In that review, Brain et al. (1988) focused primarily on the effects of genetic factors, age and nutrition, gender, smoking, and pre-existing disease states on sensitivity. Non-neoplastic and neoplastic pulmonary diseases were discussed. The analysis was limited, however, to the effects of comparatively low-concentration, long-term exposures to common air pollutants and did not provide substantial guidance relevant to short-term exposures or to the specific compounds—HCl, NO_2, and HNO_3—examined in this report.

In 1992, the World Health Organization (WHO) reviewed human health effects caused by brief episodes of air pollution and provided some information on the special needs of sensitive populations (WHO 1992). WHO stated that people with pre-existing lung disease or circulatory problems usually are more affected by episodes of increased "winter-type" (sulfur dioxide and particulates) pollution than are healthy individuals. On the other hand, for "summer-type" pollution (mostly nitrogen oxides and ozone), WHO could not identify any specific group of individuals that is more likely to be affected than other groups, although some individuals might suffer more severe responses than others.

The American Thoracic Society (ATS) analyzed the human health effects caused by air pollutants in general, including ozone, nitrogen oxides, carbon monoxide, lead, particulates, sulfur oxides, and acid aerosols (ATS 1996a,b). On balance, thorough evaluation of available epidemiological and controlled-chamber studies did not provide much evidence that adverse health effects caused by exposure to common air pollutants would be substantially more serious in potentially sensitive subpopulations (i.e., asthmatic individuals, children, and the elderly) than in the remainder of the general population.

In summary, the Brain et al. (1988), WHO (1992), and ATS (1996a,b) reports do not offer much guidance on possible safety factors or considerations that should be incorporated in exposure scenarios and risk assessments to ensure protection of sensitive subgroups. In the NRC (1993) report *Pesticides in the Diets of Infants and Children*, it was recommended that an uncertainty factor up to 10 be considered when evidence of postnatal developmental toxicity exists and when toxicity data relevant to children are incomplete.

CHEMICAL-SPECIFIC VARIATION IN HUMAN SENSITIVITY

To evaluate the potential for variation in human sensitivity to the rocket-emission toxicants specifically, the subcommittee examined data for HCl, NO_2, and HNO_3 and for two additional compounds for which extensive data on variation in human sensitivity are available—ozone and sulfur dioxide (SO_2). Data for these compounds were evaluated because the human studies allow a comparison between responses in selected groups of sensitive populations and in healthy individuals. However, the subcommittee recognizes that ozone and SO_2 are not specifically of concern to the Air Force, and the conclusions drawn from the effects of those agents cannot be assumed to apply to HCl, NO_2, or HNO_3, for which no similar data are available.

HYDROGEN CHLORIDE

Humans with respiratory problems have been presumed to be more sensitive to HCl; however, no data are available on HCl that directly support that hypothesis. Data presented in Appendix D suggest that 2 and 5 ppm might represent no-observed-effect levels (NOELs) for sensitive and healthy populations, respectively.[1] On the basis of the work of Stevens et al. (1992)—who showed that a 1.8-ppm HCl exposure to young asthmatic adults for 45 min, including two 15-min exercise periods, was without effect—2 ppm can represent a NOEL for sensitive individuals for a 45-min exposure. On the basis of general occupational experiences, industrial hygienists suggest that slight symptoms might occur at exposure concentrations around 5 ppm (see Appendix D). Thus, the human data on HCl suggest that if individuals with asthma are more sensitive, the exposure concentration associated with a threshold for response in sensitive individuals is perhaps only 2- to 3-fold lower than the concentration associated with a threshold for response in healthy individuals.

NITROGEN DIOXIDE

The data available to judge the potential impact of NO_2 on particularly sensitive subgroups are not consistent (see Appendix E). NO_2 is emitted in the home environment by gas cooking and has been reported to increase susceptibility to respiratory-tract infections in young children (Melia et al. 1979; Hasselblad et al. 1992; EPA 1993). However, that effect is believed to result from long-term exposures, which are not applicable to rocket-launch situations. Short-term exposures of human volunteers to NO_2 have generally provided conflicting results. The ATS (1996b) compiled a list of nine controlled NO_2-exposure studies of asthmatic subjects published since 1980. For seven of the studies, no changes in pulmonary function or airway responsiveness were reported. One study (Bauer et al. 1986) showed that exposure of asthmatic subjects to NO_2 at a concentration of 0.3 ppm potentiated exercise-induced bronchospasm and airway hyperactivity after cold-air provocation. By

---

[1] In this report, the phrase no-observed-effect level (NOEL) is used instead of no-observed-adverse-effect level (NOAEL) throughout because mild effects of concern to the Air Force often would not be considered adverse. Definitions of mild and adverse effects are presented in Chapter 4.

comparison, exposure of healthy humans at concentrations up to 4 ppm usually failed to affect pulmonary function (ATS 1996b). However, in another study, no significant lung-function alterations could be found in asthmatic subjects exposed at 0.3 ppm NO_2 for 1 hr (Morrow and Utell 1989). Mohsenin (1987) found heightened airway reactivity in asthmatic subjects exposed to NO_2 at 0.5 ppm for 1 hr. However, Linn et al. (1985) observed no effects in asthmatic or healthy individuals exposed to NO_2 at concentrations up to 4 ppm for 1.25 hr; that observation was attributed to potential adaptation of the subjects who lived in an area with frequent increases in common air pollutants. Morrow et al. (1992) found responsiveness to a 4-hr exposure to NO_2 at 0.3 ppm to be slightly greater in patients with chronic obstructive pulmonary disease (COPD) than in elderly healthy subjects. Interindividual variation in responsiveness also was substantially greater in elderly subjects than in the other groups (Morrow et al. 1992). Thus, some study comparisons suggest that the NO_2 concentrations at which individuals begin to respond are approximately 10-fold lower in those with asthma or COPD than in healthy individuals; other comparisons suggest no difference in the exposure concentration representing a threshold for effects in the two subgroups.

Nitric Acid

There are few human studies available for HNO_3 (Appendix F). A study by Aris et al. (1993) identified a NOEL for exposure of healthy humans to HNO_3 at 0.2 ppm for a period of 4 hr. The studies with human asthmatic subjects have shown that this portion of the population might be more sensitive to HNO_3 than healthy individuals, but the data are equivocal. Two studies by Koenig et al. (1989a,b) provide somewhat different results but suggest that some asthmatic individuals under some conditions might experience a mild, reversible increase in respiratory resistance when exposed to HNO_3 at concentrations as low as 0.05 ppm for 40 to 45 min. Applying Haber's rule to the 4-hr NOEL of 0.2 ppm for healthy adults would yield a 1-hr NOEL of 0.8 ppm, or a 45-min NOEL of 1 ppm. Comparing that NOEL with the LOEL of 0.05 ppm for individuals with asthma, both for 45 min, suggests that individuals with asthma might begin to respond at doses as much as 20-fold lower than healthy adults.

OZONE

Data are conflicting concerning the relative sensitivity of healthy adults and individuals with asthma or COPD to ozone. Several epidemiological studies strongly suggest that individuals with asthma are more sensitive to episodes of increased ozone air pollution than individuals without asthma. In controlled chamber studies, however, exposure to ozone generally resulted in only small changes or no changes in the lung function of subjects with asthma as compared with controls (Kreit et al. 1989; ATS 1996a). Similarly, the effects were not more severe in people with COPD than in people without (Linn et al. 1982; Solic et al. 1982).

SULFUR DIOXIDE

SO_2 (and sulfuric acid aerosols) can elicit more severe responses in individuals with asthma than in healthy individuals. A controlled-exposure study has shown that asthmatic subjects begin to show responses at concentrations of SO_2 (1 ppm) that are 5-fold lower than the concentrations at which healthy individuals respond (5 ppm) (Sheppard et al. 1980). In another study (Linn et al. 1987), healthy and atopic subjects showed practically no changes in pulmonary function when exposed to SO_2 at 0.6 ppm, whereas some moderately to severely asthmatic subjects responded even at 0.2 ppm, a 3-fold difference. Those asthmatic subjects responded with an increase in specific airway resistance up to 20 times higher than the healthy subjects. Those with asthma also have been found to be more sensitive to the effects of inhaled H_2SO_4 aerosols, and exposure to those aerosols is linked to increased nonspecific airway hyperactivity (Linn et al. 1989). Another function affected by inhalation of H_2SO_4 is mucociliary clearance, which usually slows in response to exposure to SO_2 (Spektor et al. 1989). That effect could be more detrimental to people with respiratory-tract infections or immunodeficiencies than to healthy individuals.

LIMITATIONS OF EXISTING STUDIES

Several limitations of the available data make it difficult to evaluate the degree to which specific human subpopulations might be more sensitive to air contaminants than healthy adults. One limitation is that most studies report only the mean values for pulmonary-function measurements; however, interindividual variation might be considerable. For example, Linn et al. (1987) reported a difference in total symptom scores of up to 10-fold or higher among moderately to severely asthmatic individuals exposed to SO_2. In fact, in an in-depth analysis of the effects of NO_2 in humans, Morrow and Utell (1989) found that among those with asthma, there appeared to be an even more-sensitive (hyperasthmatic) subpopulation.

A second limitation is that sensitive members of the population cannot be studied in a controlled setting. It is neither feasible or ethical to recruit people with severe cardiac or pulmonary disease or severe asthma into controlled exposure experiments, particularly those involving exercise. Thus, although controlled-exposure studies might confirm the suspicion derived from epidemiological studies that a more-sensitive subpopulation exists, they do not include the extremes in sensitivity that might in fact exist. It is also not feasible or ethical to conduct controlled exposure studies using infants or small children. The few epidemiological studies in which effects in children were compared with effects in adults failed to show differences (i.e., in response to acute exposures to ozone; Spektor et al. 1988; Berry et al. 1991).

A third important limitation is that studies involving human volunteers would necessarily involve exposures to comparatively low concentrations of pollutants. Because clinical studies cannot be conducted using high exposure concentrations, reliable data are lacking on the magnitude of such differences in the proportion of people affected and in the severity of response at high exposure concentrations. At higher exposure concentrations, such as those that might occur during a catastrophic abort of a rocket launch, young children or elderly people with compromised pulmonary and cardiovascular health might be disproportionately more affected than healthy individuals and show more severe responses.

Finally, experimental studies on humans measure only a few aspects of the effects of air pollution: pulmonary-function-test changes and, on occasion, minor signs of inflammatory events in airways and lung parenchyma. Such effects are considered minor and certainly not a serious threat to health, in contrast to the serious problems observed during episodes of high air pollution (i.e., increased hospital admissions and increased morbidity and mortality).

COMMON RISK-ASSESSMENT PRACTICES FOR SENSITIVE SUBPOPULATIONS

The specific issue of how to estimate risks for sensitive subpopulations was the topic of a recent symposium (Mattie 1996). An entire session was devoted to presentations discussing how to incorporate variations in human sensitivity in risk assessments. In particular, Grassman (1996) emphasized that failure to consider differences in susceptibility could result in the propagation of standards that are not protective for highly susceptible segments of the population. The subcommittee agrees in principle with that conclusion. However, Grassman (1996) used examples that cover a wide variety of disease states, from cancer to neurotoxicity, and that cover numerous individual agents. Most of those toxicants illustrate the importance of interindividual variations in metabolism and pharmacokinetics. Although the subcommittee found the information discussed in the symposium to be useful in general, it did not find any specific data relevant to the three rocket-emission compounds under consideration or to acute inhalation exposures.

In developing guidelines for setting community emergency exposure levels (CEELs) for hazardous substances, the NRC (1993) recommended consideration of the criteria for identifying sensitive subpopulations set by EPA. EPA (1994) noted that human populations, as opposed to experimental animals, react more heterogeneously to toxic agents, and defined sensitive individuals as those who experience an adverse health effect earlier or at a lower dose than the average individual. EPA (1994) recommended the use of an uncertainty factor to account for variation in sensitivity among individuals when calculating inhalation reference concentrations, intended to be safe for the general population, on the basis of data from healthy humans or animals. Specifically, the exposure concentration identified as a no-observed-adverse-effect level (NOAEL) for effects in healthy adult populations is divided by an uncertainty factor of 10 to estimate a NOAEL for potentially more-sensitive subgroups. The NRC has previously concluded that this practice is reasonable (NRC 1986, 1993, 1997). That uncertainty factor applied to a NOAEL, however, is intended to derive a "safe" exposure level (or concentration) below which adverse health effects are not expected even in sensitive subpopulations; it has no meaning for the shape or slope of the exposure-response curve. The default value of 10 is used for a wide variety of noncancer toxic end points and exposure routes, as described by Grassman (1996), not just respiratory effects resulting from an inhalation exposure.

DEFINING SENSITIVE POPULATIONS

As described in Chapter 2, the Air Force considers the sensitive subgroup to include children (less than 15 years of age), the elderly (more than 64 years of age), and all people with bronchitis, asthma, or other physiological stress, especially upper-respiratory ailments (Gene Killan, U.S. Air Force Space Command, personal commun., May 6, 1996). The subcommittee finds the phrase "physiological stress" to be too vague to be useful, is not aware of data supporting the particular age cutoffs specified, and does not support the use of age cutoffs in general for identifying sensitive subgroups. The subcommittee believes that disease state should be the principal attribute used to define sensitive subgroups. Age should be used as an attribute only to the extent that it correlates with disease states or other physiological conditions that could give rise to greater sensitivity. Selection of the exact ages for the cutoff is arbitrary and difficult to defend against claims that the age was adjusted to influence the size of the sensitive subgroup. Instead, site- and age-specific prevalence of cardiopulmonary diseases, such as asthma and COPD, together with the age distribution of the population should be used to define the sensitive subgroups; that is, in each age group (less than 15, 15 to 64, more than 64), the number of individuals estimated from U.S. Census data to be in the population near the launch site should be multiplied by the prevalence of relevant cardiopulmonary disease. The sum of those products over all age categories provides a less arbitrary (although still quite uncertain) estimate of the number of individuals in the sensitive subgroups. Where site-specific data are not available, a default prevalence from a relevant data set could be used. If it is not feasible to provide a more rigorous justification and definition of sensitive subgroups, the subcommittee questions the need for separate ERFs for sensitive and normal subgroups.

The U.S. Bureau of Census has been compiling national health data continuously since 1957. The National Health Interview Survey (NHIS) multistage probability design is intended to provide estimates of the health status of the civilian, noninstitutionalized population of the United States (Kovar and Poe 1985). Demographic and personal data collected for each survey subject include household composition, date of birth, age, sex, service in armed forces, education, race, origin, current occupation or industry, marital status, income, hospitalization history, limitation of activity, disability days, 12-month bed days, doctor contacts, general health status, height, and weight. Participants are asked questions regarding chronic health conditions of various body systems, including the skin (since 1969), the respiratory system (since 1970), and the cardiovascular system (since 1972). Conditions identified in questions concerning the respiratory-system include bronchitis, bronchiectasis, asthma, hay fever, sinus trouble, emphysema, pleurisy, tuberculosis, lung abscess, and work-related respiratory conditions. Conditions identified in questions about the cardiovascular-system include rheumatic fever, rheumatic heart disease, arteriosclerosis, congenital heart disease, coronary heart disease, hypertension, stroke or cardiovascular accident, brain hemorrhage, angina pectoris, myocardial infarction, other heart attacks, damaged heart valves, tachycardia, heart murmur, other heart trouble, and aneurysm. The subcommittee considers any of the cardiovascular and pulmonary conditions listed above as likely to render an individual more sensitive to the effects of rocket-emission toxicants than members of the population without those conditions.

CONCLUSIONS AND RECOMMENDATIONS

DEFINING SENSITIVE SUBGROUPS

Epidemiological studies strongly suggest that some individuals within any given population might be more sensitive to some air pollutants, such as NO_2, ozone, or SO_2. During episodes of heavy air pollution, most of those who seek or should get medical attention are those with asthma or the elderly suffering from COPD or other cardiopulmonary problems (ATS 1996a,b). The subcommittee recommends that disease status be used as the principal attribute for identifying sensitive subgroups rather than age cutoffs. The subcommittee believes that a more accurate assessment of the number of potentially sensitive individuals in the populations near the launch sites can be obtained by basing sensitivity on the estimated prevalence of health conditions likely to render a person sensitive rather than by basing sensitivity on indirect measurements such as age. An extensive database created by the NHIS could be used to characterize the population near launch sites by identifying the proportion of individuals in specific age categories with specific conditions that might render them more sensitive. The U.S. Census data can be used by the Air Force to obtain the age structure of the communities near launch sites.

QUANTIFYING THE DEGREE OF DIFFERENCE IN SENSITIVITY BETWEEN SENSITIVE AND NORMAL SUBGROUPS

Figure 3-1 illustrates three ways in which an exposure-versus-incidence curve for HCl, NO_2, and HNO_3 for non-immunologically mediated effects might differ between sensitive and normal populations: (1) the threshold for response for the sensitive subgroups might be lower, but the slope of the curve is similar to that for the normal population; (2) both subgroups exhibit the same threshold, but the slope of the curve for the sensitive subgroup is steeper than that for the normal population; and (3) a combination of relationships 1 and 2 also is possible. The ERFs included in LATRA assume that case 3 applies; in other words, sensitive subgroups begin to respond at lower concentrations than the normal population, and the slope of the exposure-versus-incidence curve is steeper for the sensitive subgroup than for the normal population.

Although a lower threshold and steeper slope of the exposure-versus-incidence curve for the sensitive subgroup seems reasonable, as described above, data that would allow quantifying a difference in both intercept (threshold) and slope between sensitive and normal populations are limited. There is no information for any of these toxicants relevant to the slope of an incidence-versus-exposure dose-response curve. The number of subjects included in the studies is too small, and the controlled experiments are not designed to determine how the proportion of individuals responding increases with increasing exposure concentration. There are some data relevant to the threshold for response, however. For NO_2, the data are equivocal. Some studies, but not others, suggest that individuals with asthma might begin to respond at an exposure concentration up to 10-fold lower than do normal healthy individuals. For HCl, young children or people suffering from asthma or COPD might respond at lower concentrations, but only 3-fold lower, than healthy adults. For HNO_3, the data from the few studies available

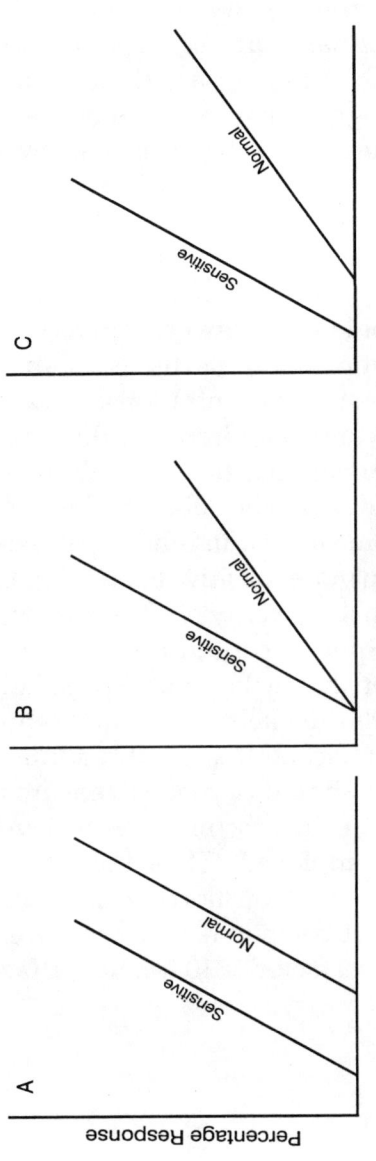

FIGURE 3-1 Hypothetical exposure-response "curves" for populations of sensitive and normal individuals. (*A*) Curves have a different intercept (threshold) but the same slope. (*B*) Curves have the same intercept (threshold) but different slopes. (*C*) Curves have a different intercept (threshold) and different slopes.

are equivocal as to whether individuals with asthma respond at lower total exposures than healthy individuals, but the difference in threshold might be as high as 20-fold.

Data from SO_2 and ozone do not show dramatic differences in sensitivity between individuals suffering from pre-existing lung diseases such as asthma or COPD and those without. Clinical studies with controlled SO_2 exposure suggest that moderately to severely asthmatic individuals might show functional changes, on average, up to 20-fold more severe than those seen in controls but that asthmatic individuals begin to respond at a concentration no more than 5-fold lower than healthy individuals. For ozone, no similar data are available, and the few studies with people suffering from COPD have shown no differences either in the threshold or severity of response.

Data for all the inhalation toxicants discussed above, however, are for comparatively low exposure concentrations. Conceivably, at higher exposure concentrations, young children or individuals with compromised pulmonary or cardiovascular health might be more *severely* affected than healthy individuals. The subcommittee concludes that, in the general population, some individuals have pre-existing conditions that are likely to make them more sensitive to NO_2, HCl, and HNO_3 than healthy individuals both in the severity of response at a given exposure concentration and in the exposure concentration and duration required to initiate a response. Given that in the general population surrounding the launch sites, individuals are likely to be found who are more sensitive to the rocket-emission toxicants than healthy adults, the subcommittee believes that provisions should be made to ensure their protection. Where the data are equivocal, the subcommittee believes that the worst-case possibility should be employed. Thus, the subcommittee recommends using the assumption that for short exposure durations (i.e., 1 hr or less), sensitive individuals begin to respond at lower concentrations than normal individuals by a factor of 10 for NO_2, a factor of 3 for HCl, and a factor of 20 for HNO_3.

4

EFFECT SEVERITY

THIS chapter presents the subcommittee's evaluation of the definition of severity categories for LATRA. In the first section of this chapter, the subcommittee reviews several precedents for severity descriptors, including the concept of severity as used by toxicologists, and the severity descriptors used by the U.S. Environmental Protection Agency (EPA) and the American Thoracic Society (ATS). The relationship between severity and sensitivity also is discussed. In the second section of this chapter, the subcommittee evaluates the LATRA model severity categories in light of those precedents. The last section provides the subcommittee's conclusions and recommendations on how severity categories can be used and how to define mild, moderate, and severe effects.

PRECEDENT FOR SEVERITY DESCRIPTORS

The concept of severity of effect is commonly used in toxicology and other health sciences. Sometimes, ratings, such as mild, moderate, and severe, are used to describe the severity of a particular outcome of exposure. In other instances, the term "adverse" is used to distinguish between outcomes that are detrimental to an organism and outcomes that are temporary physiological responses with no detrimental impact. The reversibility of an outcome is often related to severity; generally, an outcome is considered more severe if it is irreversible. The remainder of this section describes how toxicologists, EPA, and the American Thoracic Society, have used severity descriptors.

Severity of Effect in Toxicology

In toxicology, two types of dose-response curves are used (Eaton and Klaassen 1996). One type relates dose to the incidence of an effect in a group of subjects. For each subject in the group, the effect either occurs or does not occur (binary response). The second type of dose-response curve relates dose to the severity of response of an individual subject. The severity of response of a subject is "graded" according to objective or subjective criteria. Objective severity descriptors can be obtained by direct measurement (e.g., degree of cholinesterase inhibition by organophosphates). Subjective grading can be performed by an investigator, or in human experimentation, the subject might be asked to judge the severity of response. Examples of responses that often are subjectively graded are erythema and eye irritation. Toxicologists generally are referring to the second type of dose-response curve when discussing severity of effect.

Figure 4-1 illustrates the two types of dose-response curves and shows how more- and less-sensitive individuals are depicted in each type. To incorporate severity into an incidence dose-response curve, health effects would need to be categorized into discrete categories so that an individual could be classified as either showing that severity of effect or not. Figure 4-1A depicts that approach using three severity levels for coughing: mild, severe, and incapacitating. The proportion of individuals experiencing a given severity of coughing is plotted against dose. More-sensitive individuals are at the lower-left end of the curve for a specified severity of coughing, and less-sensitive individuals at the upper-right end of the curve. The curves are likely to be overlapping; some of the more-sensitive individuals might experience severe coughing at doses that only produce mild coughing in others.

For a severity dose-response curve (Figure 4-1B), severity of response is represented as a continuum. In this case, more-sensitive individuals are represented by curves starting at lower exposure concentrations, and the population is represented by a series of individual severity dose-response curves. The individual curves might be parallel (i.e., equal slopes), or the slope of the dose-response curves might be more steep for more-sensitive individuals. In either case, the severity of response in a sensitive individual would be greater than the severity of response in a normal individual at a given dose, as was shown for SO_2 in Chapter 3. The proportion of the population experiencing a given

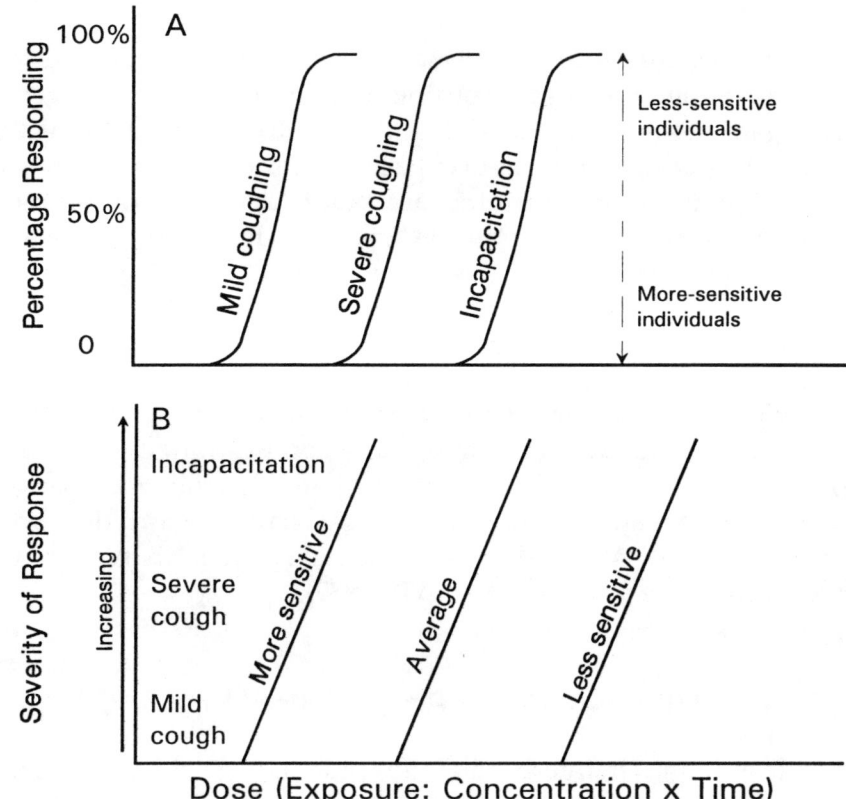

FIGURE 4-1 (A) Incidence dose-response curve. (B) Severity dose-response curve.

severity of effect at a given dose could be determined by identifying the severity level on the y-axis, the dose on the x-axis, and determining the proportion of the total number of curves representing individuals in the population that fall to the left of that point, assuming such data were available. It is more likely that a relationship between severity of response and dose would be established from a sample of individuals by regression analysis (severity of response against dose). The proportion of the population responding would be reflected in the variance of the response around the mean response predicted by the regression line. Estimating the proportion responding from that model is awkward, however, and in general, toxicologists do not use severity dose-response curves to estimate the incidence of effects.

EPA DEFINITION OF ADVERSE EFFECTS

Describing exposure effects as adverse or not adverse is a discrete severity scale for rating outcomes according to their degree of interference with an organism's normal functioning. Although carefully defining the criteria for classifying the effects of exposure to toxic substances is desirable, such severity descriptors often are loosely applied. For instance, the Clean Air Act of 1970, Section 108A, uses the term "adverse health effect" when referring to the consequences of air-pollution exposure without defining the term "adverse." To clarify this issue, EPA proposed that eye, nose, and throat irritation associated with urban smog or photochemical oxidant exposure are not medically important and, thus, should not be considered an adverse health effect (see ATS 1985). EPA developed a spectrum of biological responses ranging from the trivial to the fatal as follows: pollutant burdens, physiological changes of uncertain significance, pathophysiological changes, morbidity, and, finally, mortality. EPA considered the last three of those five categories to represent adverse responses (see ATS 1985).

AMERICAN THORACIC SOCIETY DEFINITION OF ADVERSE EFFECTS

To provide guidance in interpreting the epidemiological literature, the American Thoracic Society (ATS) defined adverse respiratory health effects as "medically significant physiologic and pathologic changes generally evidenced by one or more of the following: (1) interference with normal activity of the affected person or persons, (2) episodic respiratory illness, (3) incapacitating respiratory injury, and/or (4) progressive respiratory dysfunction" (ATS 1985). ATS also listed respiratory health effects from most severe to least severe, as shown in Appendix C.

Several aspects of the ATS discussion are particularly relevant to brief exposures, such as those possibly encountered from release of rocket propellants. First, the ATS considers certain reversible effects to be adverse. For instance, ATS considers asthmatic attacks to be adverse because they interfere with a person's normal activities, but ATS does not consider a small, brief reduction in pulmonary function to be adverse. Some measurable changes in pulmonary function due to exposure might be so slight that they are not noticeable, even for those with asthma, and ATS considers those changes to be medically insignificant.

Coughing or excess phlegm production are considered generally annoying and would be considered adverse effects only in extreme cases.

LATRA'S USE OF THE TERM "SEVERITY"

In keeping with risk estimates for other types of launch hazards of concern to the Air Force (e.g., explosions with flying debris), LATRA is designed to predict the incidence of effects, i.e., how many people would suffer an effect. To provide information to the wing commander on the seriousness of effects, the LATRA model estimates the incidence of at least mild effects and at least serious effects separately. (The definitions of mild and serious effects for LATRA are presented in Chapter 2.) Thus, in LATRA, severity of effect is incorporated in discrete categories (similar to the paradigm depicted in Figure 4-1A) rather than in a continuum from mild to severe as might be expressed by a single individual (as depicted in Figure 4-1B). In that way, the number of people likely to suffer at least a mild effect and the number of people likely to suffer at least a severe effect can be estimated.

This use of severity descriptors is fundamentally different from those used by toxicologists. In toxicology, the severity of a subject's response is graded for a single health effect (e.g., mild-to-severe coughing; see Figure 4-1B). In the LATRA paradigm, diverse potential health end points (e.g., tearing, coughing, or bronchospasm) are identified with specific severity categories. To link specific health effects with specific severity categories, the Air Force made value judgments to determine the relative significance of various health effects, but the rationale for those judgments has not been documented.

In evaluating the Air Force's use of severity descriptors, the subcommittee considered the relation between the definition of the signs and symptoms of mild and serious effects (see Chapter 2) and ATS's definition and examples of adverse effects (Appendix C). The subcommittee noted a few inconsistencies. For example, some of the responses categorized by the Air Force as severe (e.g., coughing and excess sputum) are categorized as adverse by ATS only if they are extreme. Also, many of the responses categorized as mild for LATRA are considered adverse by ATS if they either interfere with normal activities or require medical attention. Those inconsistencies point out that a specific sign, symptom, or effect by itself is not a good indicator of severity unless qualified by phrases such as "interferes with normal activities" or "requires medical attention."

CONCLUSIONS AND RECOMMENDATIONS

The subcommittee agrees that categorizing health effects into severity categories is possible and offers several advantages. The subcommittee recommends, however, a somewhat different approach to categorize effect severity than the one currently used in LATRA.

In the LATRA-ERF model, all relevant health end points are categorized as either mild or severe and grouped accordingly. That approach provides several advantages for risk communication. Those who must ultimately use the results of LATRA are not health professionals. Thus, the use of severity categories translates the risks of specific outcomes (e.g., bronchoconstriction) to more easily understood response levels (e.g., mild response). In addition, the aggregation of data for many different health end points into a few severity categories increases the amount of data available to derive each ERF relative to the amount of data available to derive an ERF for a single end point (e.g., coughing). (How the ERFs are developed for each severity category is evaluated in Chapter 5.)

The subcommittee believes, however, that effect-severity descriptors are best defined by (1) the impact on a person's ability to perform normal activities, (2) the impact on organ function, (3) the need for medical attention, and (4) the reversibility of the effect. Although some health end points are restricted to one severity category, they more often can span all severity categories. For instance, bronchochonstriction can range from mild to severe depending on its intensity. The term "adverse" has been used to describe the severity of air-pollution effects by EPA and ATS. The subcommittee has chosen not to use that descriptor because its meaning is based on the more-fundamental effect characteristics listed above.

The subcommittee recommends the following broad definitions for severity of effect for use by the Air Force. To respond to the U.S. Air Force's request for a "moderate" category in between mild and serious, the subcommittee defines three severity categories as follows. Mild effects are reversible within 48 hr and do not interfere with normal activity or require medical attention. Moderate effects are irreversible effects that do not alter organ function or interfere with normal activity, or they are reversible effects that alter organ function or interfere with normal activity. Persons experiencing moderate effects might seek medical attention. Severe effects are irreversible effects that alter organ function or interfere with normal activities. Severe effects usually require medical attention. Those definitions were developed specifically for exposures to rocket emissions and might not be applicable to other exposure scenarios or toxicants.

Table 4-1 attempts to classify the signs, symptoms, and effects of exposure of humans to rocket-emission toxicants as found in the literature into the three severity categories. Severity categories were checked if the subcommittee determined that a sign, symptom, or effect could conform to the definition of that category presented above. It is clear that many signs, symptoms, and effects cover more than one severity category and, thus, do not uniquely define the severity of an exposure outcome. Judging severity must be recognized as fundamentally a subjective process in which the values of the evaluator play a key role. Other stakeholder groups (e.g., persons living near launch areas, Air Force personnel, or individuals with asthma) might categorize these end points differently. Further difficulties with developing ERFs for severity categories are described in the next chapter. The subcommittee suggests that the Air Force be especially aware to avoid making certain value judgments based on an incomplete or limited data base. Such limitations make it difficult to evaluate or predict accurately the degree to which a specific human subpopulation might be more sensitive to air contaminants than others.

Finally, the subcommittee notes that variation in the sensitivity of individuals to toxic substances generally is accounted for in dose-response curves of the type illustrated in Figure 4-1A rather than by separate dose-response curves for more- and less-sensitive groups. That issue also is described in more detail in the next chapter.

TABLE 4-1 Classification of Potential Signs, Symptoms, and Effects of Human Exposure to Rocket-Emission Toxicants

Outcome	Mild	Moderate	Severe
Perception of odor or taste	✓		
Headache	Nonrecurring	Increased frequency	Incapacitating
Eye irritation	Discomfort	Burning sensation	
Tearing (by itself)	✓		
Corneal opacity			✓
Nasal irritation	Discomfort	Burning sensation	
Sneezing	✓		
Nasal catarrh	✓		
Rhinorrhea	✓		
Miosis	✓		
Cough	Infrequent	Frequent	Incapacitating
Burning throat			✓
Spasm of larynx			✓
Tightness in chest	✓		
Increased airway resistance	✓	✓	✓
Increased airway responsiveness	✓	✓	✓
Increased sputum production	✓	✓	
Wheezing, in absence of cold		✓	✓
Bronchospasm			✓
Sloughing of airway lining		✓	✓
Rhonchi			✓
Bronchiolitis	✓	✓	✓
Focal pneumonia	✓	✓	
Diffuse pneumonia		✓	✓
Chemical pneumonitis		✓	✓
Chest pain			✓
Shortness of breath		✓	
Difficulty breathing		✓	✓
Increase in methemoglobin	✓	✓	✓
Increase in blood pressure	✓	✓	✓
Increase in blood glutathione levels	✓		
Decrease in CO diffusion capacity	✓	✓	✓
Decrease in lung compliance	✓	✓	✓
Decrease in earlobe blood PO_2	✓	✓	✓
Decrease in alveolar O_2 partial pressure	✓	✓	✓
Pulmonary edema		✓	✓
Asthma attack	✓	✓	✓
Disorientation		✓	✓
Exacerbation of chronic cardiopulmonary disease			✓

5

EVALUATION OF THE LATRA EXPOSURE-RESPONSE FUNCTIONS

THE purpose of this chapter is to evaluate whether the forms of the ERFs used in the LATRA for HCl, NO_2, and HNO_3, are representative of the relationship between exposure and the probability of health effects. Particular attention is given to the following questions:

• What is the appropriate independent variable or variables for the ERF (maximum concentration, time-weighted-average (TWA) concentration over a defined duration, such as 5, 10, or 60 min, or the product of concentration and time)?

• What is the appropriate form of the ERF models (probit, logistic, or other)?

• What is the appropriate process for accounting for variation in sensitivity among individuals and identifiable sensitive subgroups in an exposure-response framework?

• What is the appropriate process for distinguishing among mild, moderate, and severe health effects in an exposure-response framework?

• What is the optimal process for quantifying the relation between exposure concentration and health effect using existing toxicological information on the likely incidence, sensitivity of individuals, and severity of effect?

• How should uncertainty in the estimates of risk of effects from exposure to single and multiple rocket emissions be represented in the LATRA-ERF model?

This chapter is divided into three sections. In the first section, the subcommittee evaluates the current structure of the LATRA-ERF model relative to the questions listed above. In the second section, the subcommittee suggests alternative methods for deriving ERFs that could eliminate some of the limitations in the current approach. The third section presents the subcommittee's conclusions and recommendations regarding use of the current and alternative approaches to the LATRA-ERF framework.

THE LATRA-ERF MODEL

To assess the appropriateness of the LATRA-ERF model, the subcommittee considered six issues: (1) selection of the independent variable; (2) choice of the exposure-response model; (3) representation of sensitive populations; (4) representation of severity categories; (5) selection of the chemical-specific exposure-response values to which an ERF is fit; and (6) representation and propagation of uncertainties in LATRA. During its evaluation, the subcommittee members identified a few other features of the LATRA model that they felt needed comment.

SELECTION OF INDEPENDENT VARIABLES

In the LATRA-ERF model, the independent variable for assessing health effects is the *maximum 1-hr TWA concentration* or, in some cases, *a ceiling concentration*. There are alternatives to those independent variables. The subcommittee's review of the sparse toxicity data for the compounds in question (Appendices D, E, and F) indicates that the product of concentration and time ($C \times T$) or ($C \times T^x$) appears to be a more appropriate independent variable for exposure times ranging from 5 to 60 min, at least for severe effects and mortality for HCl and NO_2 (see Chapter 6). Use of the product of exposure concentration and time as the independent variable allows estimation of the risks associated with exposures of different durations using a single ERF. With $C \times T^x$ as the independent variable for exposures from 5 to 60 min, it also is not necessary to set a ceiling concentration; the 5-min peak concentration that REEDM can estimate (it does not estimate shorter peak concentrations) is within the range of exposure durations over which the $C \times T^x$ relationship holds.

For effects for which the relationship between effect and the product of concentration and time is unknown, as might be the case for mild and moderate effects, a TWA concentration for specific exposure durations (e.g., 10 and 30 min) would be a more appropriate independent variable. The subcommittee believes that 1 hr is too long an averaging time for the exposure estimate and the toxicity value because of the typical speed with which a ground plume from a rocket launch passes over an exposure location (see Appendix A); periods of 10 to 30 min would match the exposure situation more accurately.

CHOICE OF EXPOSURE-RESPONSE MODEL

Exposure-response (or dose-response) models can be grouped into four major categories: (1) safety-factor models that estimate a safe dose for a defined population and a margin of exposure (MOE) relative to that dose (i.e., the difference between the safe dose and typical environmental exposures); (2) statistical models, such as probit or logistic models, that use observed statistical population sensitivity distributions fit to a probability distribution; (3) stochastic models, such as multihit and multistage models used for radiation- and chemical-induced cancer effects; and (4) biological-mechanism-based models. The LATRA dose-response model is intended to be a stochastic model in which the probit model represents a stochastic distribution of probability of response for a given level of severity among the population (see Chapter 2; Lloyd Philipson, ACTA Inc., personal commun., Jan. 15-16, 1997). Thus, in the LATRA model, all individuals in the population subgroup represented by the ERF are considered equally sensitive, but owing to random events, there is a probability distribution describing the likelihood of an individual suffering an effect. However, that is a departure from existing practice in toxicology in which probit or lognormal models are used to represent the variation in sensitivity to a toxic compound among individuals in a specified population.

In the LATRA-ERF model, a "safe" dose for health effects has been used in place of human data to construct the lognormal distribution, and that distribution has been interpreted as a stochastic, rather than statistical, model. That construct includes the implicit assumption that a safe exposure dose established by applying safety factors to animal or human toxicity data can be interpreted as a stochastic measurement. Because safety factors are used only to establish safe levels for healthy or sensitive populations, using safety factors to construct a stochastic exposure-response distribution goes beyond the intended use of those factors. Moreover, the LATRA ERF is reasonably interpreted as a statistical model because the probit (lognormal) function can be used to represent the variation in (or the distribution of) sensitivity among individuals in a target population. Thus, the LATRA-ERF model appears to be a hybrid between a *safety-factors* model and a *statistical* model, rather than the *stochastic* model it is stated to be.

This hybrid model introduces a problem of perception on the part of users. It suggests that the ERF is more accurate and precise than actually is true. In applying the ERF as a probit model, the user might believe (or perceive) that the model is a reliable tool for estimating the fraction of the population that is likely to experience a health effect at a given magnitude of exposure. That model is accurate, however, only when the parameters of the probit model are fit to actual exposure-versus-incidence data.

Without actual incidence data from humans or animals, it is difficult to endorse the use of exposure-response models that predict incidence of some effect type or severity, unless they are constructed using an expert elicitation process (e.g., see Evans et al. 1994). Except for the ease of use, particularly for anchoring the low and high incidence ends of the sensitivity distribution with sparse effects data, it is not clear why the probit model was used instead of other models.

Sensitive Subgroups

In theory, a probit model should be able to capture large variations among individuals in sensitivity to a toxic substance. Because the explicit purpose of a statistical model (e.g., probit model) is to construct a response function for a population with a distribution of sensitivities among the members of a population, a properly constructed probit (or logistic model) should by definition include both sensitive and healthy individuals. As a dose-response model used in toxicology, the probit model represents each individual as having a different dose at which he or she will exhibit the response.

Thus, the subcommittee considered whether the sensitive populations and healthy populations should be represented by separate ERFs or should be considered members of a single population that can be represented by a single distribution ranging from the more sensitive to the more resistant individuals (as depicted in Figure 4-1A). Historical precedent provides little assistance in answering that question; the Committee on Toxicology (COT) and other organizations generally account for subgroups likely to be more sensitive than healthy adults by applying safety factors to ensure that a threshold for response is not exceeded. There is no precedent, however, for using safety factors to estimate dose-response curves.

The most recent version of the LATRA ERFs for ceiling concentrations appears to be constructed by using a factor of 1 for HCl, 2 for NO_2, and 13 for HNO_3 to convert C_{01} ceiling concentrations (concentrations associated with a 1% response rate) for normal populations to C_{01} ceiling concentrations for the sensitive populations (see Table 2-1). (In an earlier version of the ERFs, other factors were used; Philipson et al. 1996) The toxicological bases for those three values are not clear. In the absence of data on sensitive populations, it is common practice among risk assessors to assume that the sensitive population is 10-fold more sensitive (see Chapter 3). In the past, COT concluded that it was reasonable to use factors of 2 to 10 to extrapolate between healthy and sensitive populations (NRC 1986). Data presented in Chapter 3 (and Appendices D, E, and F) indicate that the threshold for response for individuals with asthma and COPD might be lower than that for healthy individuals, on average, by a factor of 3 for HCl, 10 for NO_2, and 20 for HNO_3.

The Air Force proposes to include separate ERFs for healthy and sensitive populations so that the estimated number of people affected will be lower as the proportion of sensitive individuals in the area over which an exhaust plume is expected to pass decreases. However, with no data on how the slopes of the ERFs should differ between sensitive and normal subgroups, it is difficult to justify any particular relation between the ERF for sensitive individuals and the ERF for a healthy population beyond the relation between the concentrations associated with a threshold for response.

Another attribute of the LATRA ERFs of concern to the subcommittee is truncating the ERF at the 1% lower bound of incidence (if that value does indeed represent a 1% incidence level). The LATRA-ERF model predicts that no one is affected below the concentration associated with the 1% incidence level.

SEVERITY OF EFFECTS

In LATRA, separate ERFs were developed for different categories of severity of effect—mild and serious—rather than for specific health end points (e.g., cough or fibrosis). No clear explanation is given of how the upper-bound concentration associated with a 99% incidence of mild effects and the lower-bound concentration associated with a 1% incidence of serious effects were established for the LATRA ERFs. Ideally, the Air Force would first develop ERFs by using end points that can be clearly described (e.g., infrequent-to-moderate coughing or 20% increase in airway resistance) and then decide how to classify one or more ERFs or parts of ERFs for those specific end points into a severity category. By developing ERFs in value-based severity categories before adequate data are available, the Air Force is implicitly incorporating value judgments about severity into the ERFs in the absence of a documentable rationale. Moreover, if the Air Force were to change its valuation of the severity of different types of health effects because of a change in policy, the ERFs would have be recalculated. If ERFs were developed first by health end point, the value judgments concerning severity could be made explicit after the ERFs were fit to actual toxicity data associated with clearly described health end points.

EXPOSURE-RESPONSE VALUES

An ERF for the LATRA model is constructed by assuming that exposures considered safe correspond to 1% incidence and that the 99% incidence is 5 times the 1% incidence level for sensitive individuals and 10 times the 1% incidence level for healthy individuals (see Chapter 2). The subcommittee notes that this procedure is likely to be less accurate, possibly substantially less accurate, than fitting the ERF log-probit model to actual incidence data.

The subcommittee notes that ERFs need not be specified by symmetrical percentiles or percentiles at the extremes of the distribution. That observation is important, especially because animal and human studies seldom yield those percentiles directly. The 50th percentile is often the most precise point in a distribution, and use of *all* available data should provide the most accurate probability distribution to represent the toxicity of the agent.

In the absence of human incidence data, it might not be possible to develop accurate ERFs. Nevertheless, it should be possible to characterize the level of uncertainty associated with anchoring the probit curve by assigning a safe dose to the 1st percentile of the curve and some multiple of that to the 99th percentile. That uncertainty can be investigated through such questions as: (1) What are the appropriate percentiles to use in estimating a curve? and (2) How sensitive is the prediction of incidence to the percentiles used? One way to examine those questions is to consider an example in which several lognormal (i.e., log-probit) distributions of exposure versus the fraction of incidence have the same median value, and examine how the prediction of risk varies with the choice of percentiles used to anchor the ERF. That is done in Figure 5-1, where three ERFs for moderate effects for NO_2 are derived for healthy and sensitive populations under the assumption that the concentration at which moderate effects are seen (assumed to be 4 ppm for healthy adults and 2 ppm for sensitive populations for purposes of illustration only) correspond to the 0.1%, 1%, or 5% lower bounds of a lognormal distribution and that the upper bound of the ERF (assumed to be 40 ppm for healthy adults and 10 ppm for sensitive populations for purposes of illustration only) correspond to the 95%, 99%, and 99.9% upper bounds on the exposure-response curves. Figure 5-1 illustrates that although the central portion of the ERF is not sensitive to the assumptions regarding the incidence associated with the anchor-point concentrations, the tails are. Moreover, it is the lower tail of the distribution that is most important to the Air Force risk estimates (e.g., risk of effect of 1 in 5,000, 3 in 1,000, or 1 in 100 persons). The use of actual human incidence data would improve the accuracy of the ERF predictions.

REPRESENTATION OF UNCERTAINTIES

The subcommittee is concerned that many uncertainties in the LATRA-ERF model are not expressed or not appropriately quantified in the final model output. For example, in the procedures for applying the ERFs in LATRA, binomial distributions obtained from the $P_E(S,C,T)$ distributions are combined by adding their means and variances to obtain the mean and variance of the total number of people suffering a given severity of

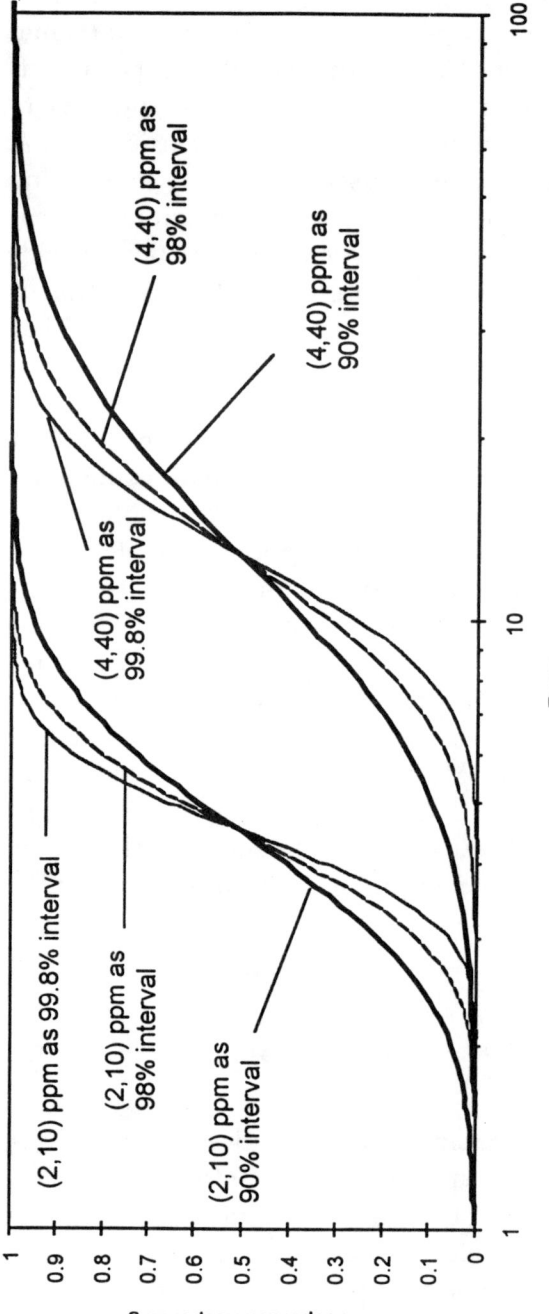

FIGURE 5-1 Sensitivity of the ERF for NO_2 to assumptions regarding interpretation of bounding values used to set cumulative distribution of the proportion of the population experiencing the effect. The curves on the left are the ERFs for sensitive populations with bounding values of 2 and 10 ppm. The heavy curve corresponds to the assumption that 2 and 10 ppm represent the 90% interval for response; 2 ppm is the concentration at which 5% of the sensitive population responds, and 10 ppm is the concentration at which 95% of the sensitive population responds. The two light curves correspond to the assumption that 2 and 10 ppm represent the 98% and 99.8% interval for response. The curves on the right are the similar ERF curves for healthy populations with bounding values of 4 and 40 ppm.

EVALUATION OF EXPOSURE-RESPONSE FUNCTIONS 53

effect at a particular receptor location. However, it is not clear to the subcommittee why the P_E function is used in a binomial to estimate the number of effects within a subpopulation. It should be recognized that

$$n(N,S,C,T) = \text{sum}(i = 1,2, \ldots N)\ \{i \times P_{\text{bnml}}[i,N,P_E(S,C,T)]\} = N \times P_E(S,C,T), \text{ i.e.,}$$
$$n(N,S,C,T) = N \times P_E(S,C,T).$$

Thus, there is no need to use the binomial distribution to estimate the expected numbers of health effects of a given severity. The variance that comes out of that approach is the variance associated with the application of the binomial to the population in a Monte Carlo simulation and excludes the variance in the function $P_E(S,C,T)$. The binomial procedure does not provide an opportunity to estimate the uncertainty in the ERFs. The binomial distribution is an appropriate distribution form for constructing a mixed distribution under Monte Carlo simulation.

The use of the binomial distribution assumes a homogenous subgroup in which every individual has exactly the same probability of developing an adverse health effect for a given exposure. Unless the subgroup is indeed homogenous, the use of the binomial distribution in this way will underestimate risk. By using the binomial model to characterize the number of effects in a finite population, the variance that results is that associated with *repeatedly* applying a model that is relevant to a large population to a small sample of that population. The subcommittee believes that this is not the appropriate variance for communicating the uncertainty associated with an ERF. The relevant variance for the ERF is the estimation error associated with fitting the log-probit model to actual exposure-response data (examples provided in Chapter 6).

OTHER FEATURES OF LATRA

The subcommittee notes that the method of estimating the potential for additive effects of simultaneous exposure to different compounds with similar modes of action in the LATRA model is likely to underestimate risks. The LATRA model simply estimates the joint probability of an effect from the independent probabilities; it does not allow for the possibility that the compounds are dose additive (i.e., exposure to subthreshold concentrations of both compounds at the same time could result in a response) or that simultaneous exposure to concentrations associated with mild responses for each compound singly could result in a severe response.

For the agents under consideration, the subcommittee is of the opinion that, in the event of a catastrophic abort when more than one of the compounds could be released simultaneously, additive effects are possible, even likely (synergistic effects are unlikely). EPA (1986) described three methods that could be used to conduct a quantitative risk assessment for mixtures of toxic substances. Their use depends on the availability of data on the mixtures and on the components of the mixtures. (A discussion of the use of these methods is in Seed et al. 1995.) The preferred method is to use data obtained from testing the actual mixture to assess the potential for health effects from exposure to the mixture. The next preferred method is to use data obtained from testing one or more mixtures with compositions similar to the mixture of interest. The third method that the EPA recommends is the component-based method, which involves assessing the risk posed by exposure to individual components of the mixture. Data from risk assessments of individual components are then used to estimate the risk from exposure to the mixture of interest by assuming a dose-additivity model for systemic toxicants and a response-additivity model for carcinogens (Seed et al. 1995). These methods have also been discussed by the NRC (1988, 1994). For the three rocket-emission toxicants reviewed in this report, it is the opinion of the subcommittee that the dose-additivity model would be appropriate.

The subcommittee is concerned with the procedure of combining risk estimates from normal launch scenarios, multiplied by the probability of a normal launch, with risk estimates from accident scenarios, multiplied by the probability of an accident, to determine the expected risk from a launch event. It is not common or accepted practice in risk assessment to combine risks for conditional events. The risks from an aborted launch are conditional on the probability of an aborted launch, and that information should be appropriately communicated in the results presented to the base commander. By combining the likelihood of a catastrophic abort and the relatively high risks associated with that event with the relatively low risks associated with a normal launch, the Air Force loses information on the event that is most likely to occur (i.e., information on risks associated with a normal launch).

It was not clear from either the technical material presented to the subcommittee or from discussions with the Air Force how the maximum 1-hr TWA concentration is selected from the output of REEDM. From the perspective of a given receptor location, the chemical concentration in the plume will first rise and then fall as the plume passes over a receptor location. It must be recognized that there are many ways to cut the resulting concentration-over-time profile into 60-min segments. It is unclear how or whether the LATRA model selects the highest 60-min concentration or ceiling concentration from the time-varying concentration at a given location.

Many of the ERFs have very steep slopes, ranging from essentially zero incidence to 100% incidence over roughly an order of magnitude change in concentration. Given that atmospheric models can at best only predict concentrations within a factor of 2 or 3 at a single location (Turner 1994), the subcommittee is concerned about the reliability of the overall process with such models for estimating incidence of health effects in exposed populations.

ALTERNATIVE APPROACHES

As discussed in Chapters 3 and 4, dose-response curves are used to provide two types of information — (1) the relationship between dose and incidence of effect in a group of subjects and (2) the relationship between dose and severity of effect. Most dose-response models provide only one of those relationships but not both. The LATRA-ERF model is designed primarily to provide incidence data. As part of the process for evaluating the LATRA-ERF, the subcommittee explored the capabilities and limitations of a number of alternate approaches to the current LATRA-ERF model. Particular attention was given to approaches that include both severity and incidence information in a single model, such as ordinal regression. The results of those evaluations are summarized in this section.

GENERAL CONSIDERATIONS IN DOSE-RESPONSE MODELS

The purpose of the LATRA ERF is to provide a model that links the expected number and severity of effects with both exposure concentration and exposure duration. There are a number of alternative formulations for defining this relationship—ranging from simple threshold models to complex multiple regression models. Model selection depends on the quantity and quality of the available data.

In the most general sense, the subcommittee considered a model of the form

$$P(Y \geq S|C,T) = \text{function }(Y,S,C,T),$$

where $P(Y \geq S|C,T)$ is the ERF for an exposure characterized by concentration, C, and time, T, and is equal to the probability of the severity of effect, Y, equaling or exceeding a given severity category, S, at a specified exposure concentration, C, and duration T.

The simplest form of this model, based on the use of a single population threshold, is

$$P(Y \geq S|C,T) = 1 \text{ when } C > \text{threshold }(T,Y) \text{ and } = 0 \text{ otherwise.}$$

The next level of complexity would give a simple probit model:

$$P(Y \geq S|C,T) = O(A + B \times C) \text{ for each } Y \text{ and } T \text{ (5, 10, 60 min etc.);}$$

or a more complex probit model:

$$P(Y \geq S|C,T) = O[A + B \times (CT^g)] \text{ for each } Y.[2]$$

Setting $g = 1$ would result in a strict Haber's rule model. Haber's rule states that the biological effects of some types of toxicants tend to be related to the total cumulative exposure (area under the concentration-time curve). For a strict Haber's rule model, the total exposure for risk estimation is the TWA concentration (C) multiplied by the time (T) (duration of exposure).

Another model at this level of complexity would be a logistic model, which would take the form

$$P(Y \geq S|C,T) = \exp[A + B \times (CT^g)]/\{1+ \exp[A + B \times (CT^g)]\} \text{ for each } Y.$$

With the same data (i.e., the same 1% and 99% bounds), the probit and

---

[2] O designates the cumulative normal distribution.

the logistic models give similar results in the 1% to 99% incidence range. However, these two models give significantly different results outside the data range for which they are calibrated. The logistic model is more flexible in handling exposure concentration versus time. Figure 5-2 compares the predictions of the two models for estimating an ERF for NO_2.

ORDINAL REGRESSION

Ordinal regression is an example of a more comprehensive and flexible approach for relating both incidence and severity of effects to both exposure concentration and duration. Ordinal regression was first proposed by Hertzberg and Miller (1985) and later was refined by Guth et al. (1991). In this approach, health effects are first assigned to severity categories based on evaluation of the reported information and consideration of biological and statistical significance. The aggregate group of subjects at any particular exposure concentration and duration is classified as giving evidence of a specific severity of response. A model, such as the logistic regression model, is applied using the severity code as the dependent variable and the exposure concentration and exposure duration as the independent variables. For any level of severity, the output of the regression provides a concentration-by-duration profile (both central estimates and confidence-limit estimates) for any desired risk level.

The ordinal regression model continues to be refined and applied to some specific chemicals and data (Simpson et al. 1996), but the data requirements and complexities of the model fitting make the model infeasible for routine use or use in LATRA. The available toxicity data for HCl, NO_2, and certainly for HNO_3, include few or no studies with dose-response data for non-lethal effects. Ordinal regression also requires that levels of severity are assigned to effects data prior to developing the regression model. Any changes in interpretation of the severity of various signs or symptoms would require that the ordinal regression model be recalculated. Finally, in this method, the imprecision of the estimate of the probability of an effect in a given severity level is reflected in the confidence-limit estimate for the central tendency. Thus, a statistical refinement of the LATRA model would be required to derive estimates of the risk or incidence of individuals suffering an effect of at least a given severity level.

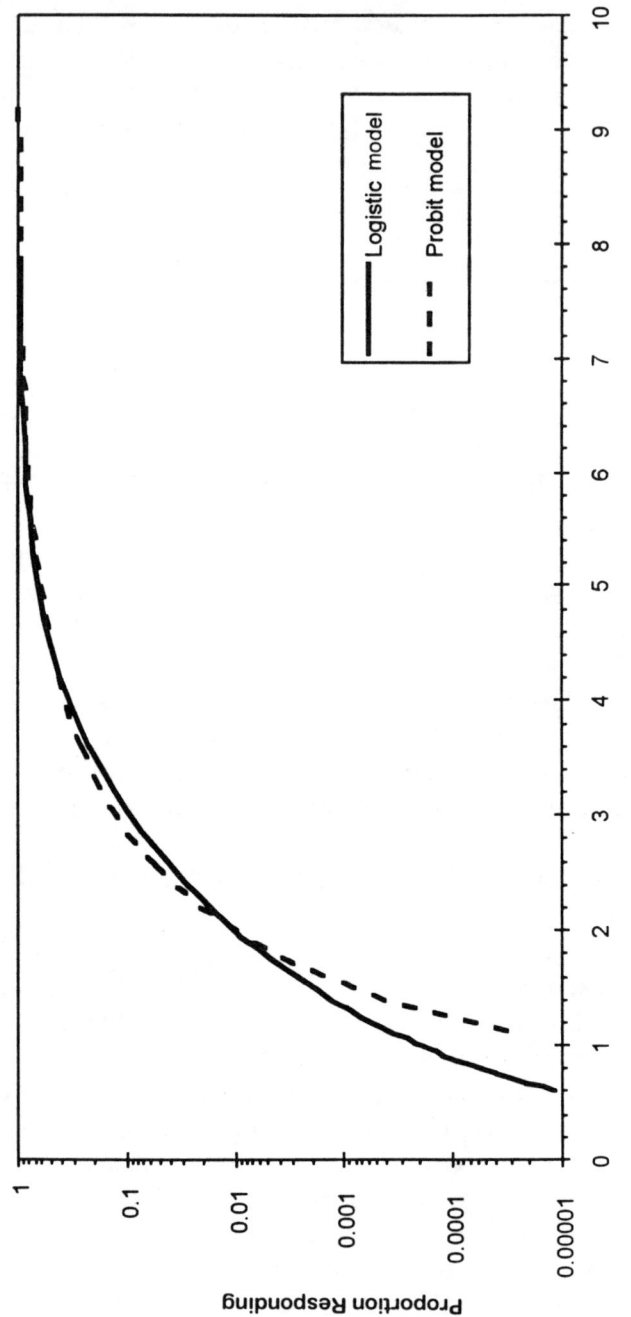

FIGURE 5-2 Sensitivity of the ERF for NO_2 to the dose-response model. The two dose-response curves for the sensitive population correspond to the assumption that 2 ppm results in a 1% incidence and 10 ppm results in a 99% incidence. The two dose-response models are similar in their predictions down to an exposure of about 2 ppm. Below that concentration, the logistic model gives a higher fraction of response at a given concentration of exposure. At 1 ppm, the fraction of response predicted by the two models differs by more than an order of magnitude.

MAXIMUM ENTROPY INFERENCE

The maximum-entropy-inference (MEI) method uses subjectivity to develop distribution functions with sparse data (Lee and Wright 1994). Entropy, in its strictest definition, is a tendency toward disorder. When an attempt is made to maximize the entropy of a distribution, conclusions are made about the data but made in a way that is inclusive of all variance — both variance associated with variability (due to inherent randomness in the observed populations) and variance associated with uncertainty (due to measurement error, observation error, or lack of knowledge). The entropy of a distribution, H, is defined as a measure of its uncertainty. The method requires a constraint and maximizes the uncertainty of the model distribution given that constraint. Examples of constraint are a range limitation (minimum and maximum values), a bound on the median or mean, or a constraint on some other characteristic of a distribution including a variance value or percentile values. In a certain sense, the MEI method chooses a shape, given what is known (i.e., the constraints), that provides a maximum spread of information with a minimum chance of any plausible outcome being excluded from the range of outcomes produced. This method is only as biased as the methods used to estimate the constraints. It requires, however, knowledge of the scale at which the data are distributed; it must be decided whether to maximize the uncertainty in the units of the data or in the transformed state (e.g., log transform). The method provides a distribution that maximizes H, given the entropy is calculated as

$$H = \int p(x) \log_2 p(x) dx$$

for continuous distributions. If the Air Force wishes to pursue the development of ERFs further, it would be appropriate for it to consider whether the MEI approach would be useful for characterizing the uncertainty in the exposure-response relationship.

HAZARD-QUOTIENT–HAZARD-INDEX APPROACH

The hazard-quotient model is simply a comparison of the estimated exposure concentration (EEC) to a NOEL or other reference toxicity

> **Hazard-Index (HI) Calculation**
>
> $HI = EEC_1/RTV_1 + EEC_2/RTV_2 + \ldots + EEC_i/RTV_i$
>
> *where* EEC_i = estimated environmental concentration for the ith contaminant;
>
> *and* RTV_i = reference toxicity value (e.g., a NOEL) for the ith contaminant.
>
> Individuals for which the HI > 1 are assumed to be at risk of a an effect from exposure to the combination of contaminants.
>
> The EEC and RTV values should be expressed in the same way. Thus, if the RTV is expressed as exposure concentration multiplied by time (C × T), the EEC should also be in units of C × T; if the RTV is a function of C for a specified duration, the EEC should be expressed as a concentration for that exposure duration.

value (RTV) (e.g., threshold for moderate effects). The Air Force's comparison of its tier limits to the exposure concentrations estimated by REEDM is an example of the hazard-quotient model. Usually, the RTV is developed so that it is a conservative estimate of a threshold concentration (or dose) above which some health effects might occur in some individuals and below which, effects are considered unlikely to occur in most or all individuals in a specified group or population. Thus, when the ratio of the EEC to the RTV is less than 1 (i.e., the quotient EEC/RTV is less than 1), effects are considered unlikely. When the quotient is greater than 1, some effects might occur in some individuals. Interpretation of the ratio of the two values depends on the uncertainty associated with each. As the value of the EEC/RTV increases, both the severity and incidence of effect are likely to increase, but the ratio is not used to predict incidence or severity.

Estimating the number of people exposed at levels above RTVs using the hazard-quotient model would not produce risk estimates that are more precise or accurate than the available toxicity data would warrant. RTVs can be developed to represent no-observed-effect levels (NOELs) or thresholds for mild, moderate, and severe effects. In a risk assessment, the magnitude of an EEC/RTV estimate also can be useful information to a risk manager, even though that value cannot be related to incidence or severity of effect. An additional advantage of the hazard-quotient model is that it allows estimation of the number of people at risk of additive effects from simultaneous exposure to two or more substances, a consideration that is not appropriately represented in the LATRA model and that would be difficult to develop in the ERF framework.

To apply dose-additivity to the hazard-quotient approach, it is only necessary to sum the hazard quotients for the individual emission toxicants (see text box). That sum is commonly called the hazard index (EPA 1989). A hazard index should be estimated separately for each exposure duration or C × T modeled. A risk of a health effect is assumed to exist at
those exposure locations where the hazard index exceeds 1. As was the case for the individual hazard quotients, interpretation of hazard indices greater than 1 depends on the assumptions inherent in the estimate of exposure and estimate of a NOEL or other RTV, and hazard indices cannot be associated with incidence of effects.

CONCLUSIONS AND RECOMMENDATIONS

Overall the subcommittee does not endorse use of the LATRA-ERF model as it currently is constructed. The ERFs give the appearance of substantial accuracy, yet are not supported by the available toxicological information. The subcommittee suggests, as a possible alternative, application of the hazard-quotient–hazard-index approach to risk characterization for the rocket-emission toxicants. However, if the Air Force wants to pursue the LATRA-ERF model (e.g., using expert elicitation to establish ERFs), there are ways to improve that framework. The subcommittee's conclusions and recommendations regarding each of the six issues are described below. A few recommendations on other features of LATRA also are provided.

SELECTION OF THE INDEPENDENT VARIABLE

The ERFs in LATRA are currently based on 1-hr TWA concentrations and ceiling values. The subcommittee believes that 1 hr is too long an averaging period because of the typical speed with which the ground cloud of emissions from a rocket launch pass over a given exposure location; increments of 10 to 30 min would match the exposure situation more accurately. The subcommittee endorses the use of ceiling values for noncumulative effects. The subcommittee also identified some effects for which the product of exposure concentration and time ($C \times T$) would be appropiate. It recommends that sensitivity of the LATRA output to the selection of the independent variable be examined. The evaluation should include how the estimates of the number of health effects in a given category of severity (e.g., mild or severe) depend on (1) which independent variable (the TWA concentration or the total cumulative exposure) is used and (2) which averaging time is used to estimate the TWA concentration in the ERF. If the TWA concentrations for 10, 30, and 60 min are used, those results should be compared with the results of using total cumulative exposure ($C \times T$ or the time integral of concentration).

CHOICE AND QUANTIFICATION OF EXPOSURE-RESPONSE MODEL

A log-probit model is an appropriate analytic form for a dose-response model that will be used to estimate incidence of effects. A key weakness of the current derivation of LATRA ERFs, however, is that a dose-response model for predicting incidence is derived from concentrations that are used to define safe levels (at the lower bound) and dangerous levels (at the upper bound). The subcommittee does not believe that it is appropriate to assume that no health effects occur below a 1% incidence level for mild effects. Nor does the subcommittee believe that it is appropriate, in the absence of supporting data, to interpret a concentration that is 5- or 10-fold higher than a 1% incidence level as the concentration at which all individuals are likely to show those responses. More important, combining two such values to construct a model for predicting incidence in the range between those values lacks support from either epidemiological or toxicological data. In short, the concentrations that are used have no specified relation to incidence and thus should not be used as predictors of incidence without explicit explanation of the unknown accuracy of such an approach.

To the extent possible, the Air Force should use end-point-specific incidence data to develop end-point-specific ERFs. However, with the exception of mortality and a few other end points, incidence data for HCl, NO_2, and HNO_3 are not available (see Appendices D, E, and F and Chapter 6). Without incidence data from humans or animals, it is difficult to endorse the use of exposure-response models that predict incidence unless they are constructed through some type of expert elicitation process. In such a process, a group of selected experts would be interviewed using carefully developed procedures to elicit their individual professional opinions concerning what health effects would be expected at each of a series of exposure durations and concentrations. Their opinions would be compared by a formal process, and a majority opinion and the range in opinions would be used to establish a quantitative relationship between exposure and effect and the uncertainty of opinion concerning that relationship. For an example of a properly constructed expert elicitation process, see Evans et al. (1994).

Until more data become available or such an expert elicitation can be carried out for end points with no incidence data, the subcommittee believes that a hazard-quotient model would be more appropriate. For the hazard-quotient model, estimates of the number of people at risk would be based on the number of people with exposures above a no-observed-effect level. How far exposure concentrations are above safe levels might also be useful information. The hazard-quotient model also could be used to estimate how many people might be at risk of moderate or severe effects if the Air Force is willing to accept the level of uncertainty associated with the exposure values identified as thresholds for moderate and severe effects (see Appendices D and E).

SENSITIVE SUBGROUPS

Under the LATRA model, separate ERFs are developed for sensitive and normal populations. However, a properly constructed probit model can portray wide variation in human sensitivity within a single exposure-response function. Moreover, available data are insufficient to quantify different ERFs for sensitive and healthy (normal) populations. Thus, the subcommittee cannot support the use of separate ERFs for sensitive and normal populations, although it does support the use of different thresholds for effect if the hazard-quotient–hazard-index approach is used to characterize risk.

Under the LATRA model, the ERFs are truncated at the 1% incidence level, which suggests that there are no effects at lower exposure concentrations. In a true probit or logistic model, a small but still significant probability of incidence occurs below the 1% level. With a large nearby population, dozens of people could be affected at or below the exposure concentrations associated with a 1% incidence level. Using actual incidence data to construct the ERF would make it possible to predict the incidence below the 1% level. In the absence of incidence data to construct ERFs, however, this issue is not of concern.

SEVERITY OF EFFECTS

To avoid embedding value judgments in the scientific exposure-response analysis, the subcommittee recommends that, if ERFs are used, they be developed first by health end point. Then decisions can be made as to which exposure concentrations to associate with mild, moderate, and severe effects, considering all end points and variation in severity within end points (e.g., mild to severe bronchoconstriction). However, incidence dose-response data are lacking for all but severe end points for HCl and NO_2 and are altogether lacking for HNO_3. It is possible to estimate a threshold for mild effects (based on a NOEL). It also might be possible to estimate thresholds for moderate and severe effects for HCl and NO_2 (see Appendices D and E), although there are large uncertainties associated with the time-dependence of those estimates. Those thresholds could be used with the hazard-quotient approach to characterize risk.

REPRESENTATION AND PROPAGATION OF UNCERTAINTIES

Uncertainties in LATRA predictions arise from a number of sources, including specification of the problem; formulation of the conceptual model and the computational model; estimation of input values; and calculation, interpretation, and documentation of the results. Of those sources, only uncertainties due to estimation of input values can be quantified in a straightforward manner based on the type of variance propagation techniques used in the LATRA-ERF model. However, the LATRA model does not formally address the uncertainties and variability in the air concentrations of exposures derived from LATRA. In addition, uncertainties that arise from misspecification of the problem and model-formulation errors generally are not assessed in LATRA.

With regard to uncertainties in the LATRA process, the subcommittee observes that the use of complex stochastic simulations of exposure response cannot be justified when the underlying toxicological data are inadequate or essentially absent, as is the case for the compounds of interest in this study. In this situation, a formal stochastic analysis can obscure the important source of uncertainty—the absence of complete toxicological data. The absence of concentration-response data can be remedied by the collection of more data, particularly data that can be used to assess variation in susceptibility in human populations. Until such data become available, ERFs that express variability of response cannot be constructed.

The binomial model generates a variance that underestimates the variance associated with fitting the ERF to response data. The subcommittee recommends not using the binomial model in LATRA to assess uncertainty. Variability and uncertainty in the distribution of health outcomes should be retained in reporting the final results across different population subgroups and rocket-emission release scenarios.

It is recommended that sensitivity analyses be conducted to investigate the impact of the assumptions and procedures used to construct the ERFs on the model predictions of risk. It is also recommended that the Air Force generate appropriate toxicity data to calibrate and validate the proposed model. The investments in appropriate testing procedures, at this time, would be worth the effort by improving the model predictibility and reducing the uncertainty. Such studies should, at a minimum, examine concentration times, time responses, and include adequate histopathology. This will allow the Air Force to calibrate their model more appropriately based on sound data.

OTHER FEATURES OF LATRA

The subcommittee recommends that the Air Force evaluate potential health effects resulting from simultaneous exposure to more than one toxic rocket emission assuming the potential for additive effects. That could be accomplished using the hazard-index approach to characterize risk.

Instead of presenting one risk estimate for a launch, combining the risks of a normal launch and catastrophic abort, the subcommittee believes that it would be appropriate for the Air Force to present risks for the normal and aborted launches separately or to provide both separate conditional risks and combined risks.

The Air Force should ensure that any TWA exposure estimates used to estimate risk are the maximum values possible for that averaging time. For example, the maximum 30-min concentration passing over an exposure location should be the value compared with a 30-min ERF or effect threshold.

The subcommittee also recommends that the Air Force evaluate the relative accuracies of the exposure estimates from REEDM and the ERFs (or effect thresholds suggested here). If the Air Force can determine whether it is the exposure or effects component of LATRA that is the more serious limit to the model's accuracy in predicting risk, it can invest efforts in improving the less accurate component.

6

EXPOSURE-RESPONSE FUNCTIONS FOR ROCKET-EMISSION TOXICANTS

THIS chapter provides examples of procedures for developing ERFs for the three rocket-emission toxicants — HCl, NO_2, and HNO_3 — according to the subcommittee's recommendations in Chapter 5. The ERFs are derived from available exposure-response data for those compounds, rather than set by simply estimating the exposures associated with a 1% and a 99% incidence on a lognormal distribution, as is currently done for the LATRA-ERF model. As will become clear in this chapter, few health end points have sufficient data to estimate ERFs for the rocket-emission toxicants.

This chapter is organized in five sections. The first three sections provide analyses of quantal exposure-response data for the three rocket-emission toxicants in order of increasing data availability — HNO_3, HCl, and NO_2. The fourth section provides an example of how to develop an ERF from continuous, instead of quantal data, using data from toxicity studies of NO_2. The final section presents the subcommittee's conclusions and recommendations regarding use of these ERFs in LATRA.

NITRIC ACID

An acute toxicity profile for nitric acid (HNO_3) is provided in Appendix F. HNO_3 can produce respiratory damage because it is a strong acid, it is an excellent oxidizing agent, and it reacts immediately with any tissue it contacts. It causes such effects as skin burns, eye irritation, coughing, dyspnea, and pulmonary edema. The serious respiratory effects, including pulmonary edema, can occur several hours after an acute exposure and are probably related to inflammation resulting from cellular necrosis in lung tissues.

Several studies have shown that exposure to HNO_3 at concentrations up to 0.2 ppm for 4 hr produces no observable effects in healthy humans. Concentrations as low as 0.05 ppm might cause some mild respiratory effects in asthmatic individuals. The subcommittee estimates that a no-effect level for HNO_3 is 1.0 ppm (ceiling) for periods up to 1 hr for healthy individuals and 0.05 ppm (ceiling) for periods up to 1 hr for asthmatic individuals and others with compromised respiratory function. However, as described in the following subsections, an exposure-response function (ERF) cannot be established for HNO_3 in healthy individuals or in asthmatic individuals, because too few data have been published on the effect levels of HNO_3 for animals or humans.

HEALTHY ADULTS

The no-observed-effect level (NOEL) for humans exposed to HNO_3 is 0.2 ppm for 4 hr (Aris et al. 1993) (see Chapter 3 and Appendix F). In that study, 10 persons were exposed and examination by bronchoscopy 18 hr later, revealing no adverse effects. If Haber's rule applies, an acceptable exposure concentration is 0.8 ppm (i.e., 0.2 ppm × 4) for 1 hr and 1.6 ppm for 30 min. Those concentrations are based on observing no effects in 10 individuals. When a small number of subjects are used (10 in this case), little confidence can be placed in the observation of no effects, and a confidence limit should be calculated for the observation. The true probability of an observable effect at a concentration of 0.2 ppm for 4 hr could be as high as 0.067, with a 50% chance of observing no effects in 10 individuals. That is, the probability of not observing an effect in 10 individuals is $(1 - 0.067)^{10} = 0.50$. That calculation provides a means of obtaining a conservative risk estimate even though no responses occurred in a small sample. If the probability of an observable effect is 0.067 at 0.2 ppm for 4 hr, and if Haber's rule applies, an exposure at 0.8 ppm for 1 hr implies the same risk of 0.067, or an incidence of 67 per 1,000 individuals. Thus, an incidence of 0.067 at a contamination of 0.8 ppm for 1 hr is one data point that might be used in establishing an ERF.

Abraham et al. (1982) exposed seven normal sheep to HNO_3 vapor at a concentration of 1.6 ppm for 4 hr. "Two of the normal sheep responded with large post-HNO_3 exposure increases in air reactivity"; increases were over 100% in specific airway resistance of the lung. Those data indicate a risk of 2/7 (0.29) at a concentration of 1.6 ppm for 4 hr. If Haber's rule applies, an exposure at 6.4 ppm for 1 hr implies a risk of 0.29. That provides a second data point for developing an ERF, assuming that sheep and humans respond similarly to HNO_3.

For the healthy adult population, only the two data points described above are available to establish an ERF for HNO_3. Both points are based on a small sample size, both depend on Haber's rule, and the second data point is based on animals, not humans. Thus, the subcommittee believes that an ERF for respiratory resistance based on those two data points is too uncertain to estimate human health risks associated with exposure to HNO_3. Using the hazard-quotient approach to estimating the number of individuals who might be exposed at concentrations above a NOEL would be an appropriate alternative (see Chapter 5).

SENSITIVE SUBJECTS

Koenig et al. (1989a) obtained measurements on adolescent asthmatic subjects exposed to HNO_3 at a concentration of 0.05 ppm for 40 min. One of seven subjects showed an increase in respiratory resistance of 70% (see Appendix F). If Haber's rule applies, then 0.033 ppm for 1 hr corresponds to a risk of increased respiratory resistance of 1/7 (or 14%). A later study, however, showed no effects (Koenig et al. 1989b). Thus, a risk of 14% at 0.033 ppm for 1 hr could serve as a conservative estimate of one of the two points needed to develop an ERF for individuals with asthma. Abraham et al. (1982) reported that six of seven hypersensitive sheep exposed to HNO_3 at 1.6 ppm for 4 hr showed increases of over 100% in specific airway resistance of the lung. Those data indicate a risk of 6/7 (86%) at 1.6 ppm for 4 hr. If Haber's rule applies, an exposure at 6.4 ppm (i.e., 1.6 ppm × 4) for 1 hr implies a risk of 86%, which could be used as a second point to establish an ERF for sensitive individuals. This assumes that hypersensitive sheep and sensitive humans respond similarly to HNO_3.

Based on the above data, sensitive individuals might be 20 times more sensitive than healthy individuals at low concentrations of HNO_3, as stated in Chapter 3. However, as indicated for healthy individuals, the subcommittee believes that an ERF for respiratory resistance for sensitive individuals based on only two data points (with small sample sizes, using Haber's rule, and with the second point based on animal data) is too uncertain to estimate the incidence of effects associated with exposure to HNO_3 from rocket launches.

HYDROGEN CHLORIDE

An acute toxicity profile for hydrogen chloride (HCl) is provided in Appendix D. HCl is a highly irritating gas or aerosol, depending on environmental exposure conditions. The toxicity of the gas and aerosol are similar in animal studies. The toxicity of HCl in humans and animals is related to its surface-damaging properties. Therefore, the mechanism of action of HCl in animals and humans is expected to be similar. Although damage to the upper respiratory system and eyes is possible from exposure to HCl, serious damage to these structures is only seen at high exposure concentrations. Of more concern is inhalation of HCl into the airways of the lower respiratory system at high exposure concentrations. The few studies on adults with mild asthma suggest that asthmatic individuals might not be more susceptible to low concentrations of HCl than nonasthmatic individuals. However, as the protective properties of the upper airways are overcome, those with asthma might show significantly greater sensitivity to HCl.

Data presented in Appendix D suggest that 2 and 5 ppm might represent no-observed-effect levels (NOELs) for sensitive and healthy populations, respectively. There are no data by which to estimate ERFs for HCl for mild effects for sensitive or healthy populations.

Dose-response incidence data are available for HCl for two end points only: mortality and corneal opacity (see Appendix D). ERFs can be developed for those end points as described below. It is unlikely, however, that ERFs for those endpoints would be useful to the Air Force. They are presented primarily to show how ERFs can be developed from quantal dose-response (incidence) data.

MORTALITY

Data on rodent mortality provide the most information available for establishing ERFs for HCl. Because mice are more sensitive than rats to HCl (see Appendix D), ERFs for mice were developed. However, it must be kept in mind that mice are also more sensitive than humans to HCl (Appendix D).

Darmer et al. (1974) exposed mice for 5 or 30 min at several concentrations of HCl. Mortality is plotted in Figure 6-1 on log-probability (log-probit) scales. The linear plots indicate that the logarithm of fatal concentrations is reasonably well described by a normal distribution (i.e., a lognormal distribution). The 30-min exposure is about six times more potent than the 5-min exposure, indicating that Haber's rule applies to the mortality end point for those concentrations and durations of exposure. Because Haber's rule applies and the studies by Darmer et al. (1974) and Wohlslagel et al. (1976) have similar results, the 5- and 30-min mortality results are plotted in Figure 6-2 as a single ERF for percentage dead versus cumulative (total) exposure, which is expressed in milligram-minutes per cubic meter.

No deaths occurred in two groups of animals in those experiments

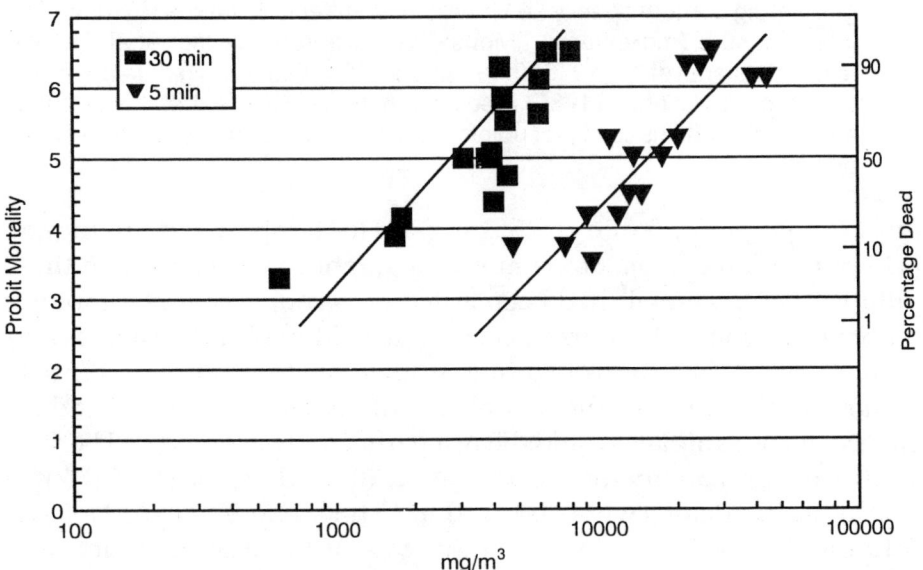

FIGURE 6-1   Plots (log-probit) of mouse mortality (percentage dead) versus HCl exposure concentration (mg/m^3) for 30 min (■) and 5 min (▼). Data are from Darmer et al. (1974) (see Appendix D). See text of this chapter for percentages used to plot points representing groups of animals in which all or no animals died.

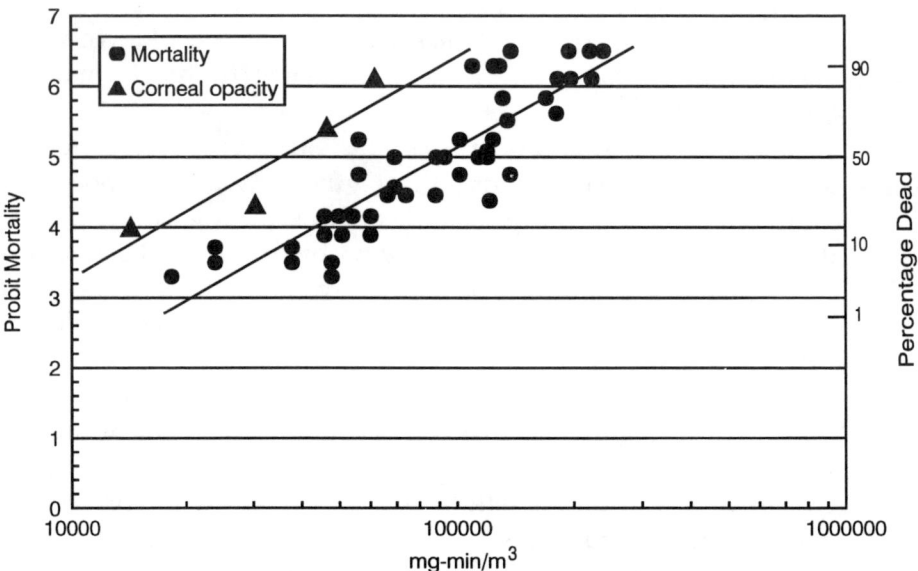

FIGURE 6-2 Plots (log-probit) of mouse mortality (●) (percentage dead) and guinea-pig corneal opacity (▲) (percentage affected) versus HCl cumulative exposure (mg•min/m^3). Mouse data are from Darmer et al. (1974) and Wohlslagel et al. (1976) (see Appendix D). Guinea-pig data are from Burleigh-Flayer et al. (1985) (see Appendix D). See text of this chapter for percentages used to plot points representing groups in which all or no animals died.

(group exposed for 5 min at 9,551 mg/m^3 (6410 ppm) and 610 mg/m^3 (410 ppm) (Table D-6). Some mortality might have occurred in those groups if more animals had been tested per group. That possibility is particularly true for the 5-min exposure at 9,551 mg/m^3, because deaths occurred in other groups exposed at lower concentrations. With 10 animals in a group, the true mortality could be as high as 0.067 and the chance that no animals would die in a particular test would still be 50%. That is, the probability that no animals in 10 would die is $(1 - 0.067)^{10} = 0.50$. Also, no deaths were observed in 15 mice exposed to 610 mg/m^3 (410 ppm) of HCl for 30 min. In this case, if the true mortality were 0.045, there is a 50% chance that no deaths would occur in a sample of 15 animals. The 50% confidence limits are the incidences plotted in Figures 6-1 and 6-2 for those two groups where no mortality was observed.

In three other groups of animals, mortality was 100%; however, if more animals had been included in those groups, some might have survived. Thus, the true mortality could be as low as 93.3%, and the chance of obtaining a 100% mortality of 10 animals would still be 50%. That percentage is a conservative adjustment for the ERF at low concentrations of HCl, because it lowers the slope of the ERF and, in turn, increases the incidence of effects at the low exposure concentrations. Such adjustments provide a conservative correction for potentially unlikely results that are due to small sample sizes.

Because the variation in response rate with exposure is relatively constant across exposure concentration multiplied by time, a simple least-squares fit is applied to the mouse mortality data (Figure 6-2), giving

$$\text{probit} = -10.59 + 1.366 \ln(CT),$$

where C is concentration in milligrams per cubic meter and T is duration in minutes. The ERF for mortality in mice shown in Figure 6-2 is relatively steep. Mortality changes from 5% to 95% over a 12-fold increase in the total exposure. The HCl exposure estimated to correspond to a risk of 10^{-4} (probit = 1.28) is 5,940 mg•min/m^3 (3,990 ppm•min).

The Air Force does not include lethality in its LATRA risk assessment for rocket-launch emissions. If the Air Force wanted to estimate the possibility that someone might die from emissions from a rocket launch, it could use the mouse model as a conservative estimate, because the mouse is the most sensitive of the animal species tested for acute effects (Appendix D). Humans can be expected to have responses to HCl that are more like those of baboons because the upper respiratory tract of the baboon is most like that of humans, and the geometry of the upper respiratory tract is expected to play an important role in moderating the toxicity of inhaled HCl. Because the sensitivity to HCl is greater in mice than baboons and assuming humans have responses to HCl which are more like baboons, no additional safety factor is needed, and the mouse model is likely to overestimate risks of death in humans. Because only a few thousand people are likely to be exposed to substantial amounts of HCl under the worst conditions, the mouse model indicates that a total exposure of 3,990 ppm•min is unlikely to result in any human deaths. Over a 60-min interval, the average concentration is 66 ppm (3,990 ppm•min/60 min). Applying Haber's rule, the average concentrations that are unlikely to result in any human deaths for 60-min or less are shown below.

Duration (min)	HCl (ppm)
60	66
30	130
10	400
5	800

CORNEAL OPACITY

Corneal opacity resulting from HCl exposure was observed in guinea pigs by Burleigh-Flayer et al. (1985); the NOEL was 320 ppm (477 mg/m^3) for 30 min (Appendix D). The true risk of corneal opacity could be as high as 15.9% with a 50% chance of not observing any such effects in four animals. That incidence was plotted in Figure 6-2 and was used in curve fitting. Also, the incidence of corneal opacity at 1,380 ppm (2,056 mg/m^3) was adjusted from 100% to 87.1%, because the incidence could be that low with a 50% chance that all five animals would exhibit corneal opacity. The least-squares line for corneal opacity was

$$\text{probit} = -9.957 + 1.425 \ln(CT),$$

where C is concentration in milligrams per cubic meter and T is duration of exposure in minutes.

The exposure estimated to correspond to a risk of corneal opacity in guinea pigs of 10^{-4} (1 in 10,000) was 2,660 mg•min/m^3 (1,785 ppm•min). Using Haber's rule, exposures that are not likely to result in severe effects, such as corneal opacity observed in guinea pigs, are shown below.

Duration (min)	HCl (ppm)
60	30
30	60
10	180
5	360

DOSE-RESPONSE FOR MILD, MODERATE, AND SERIOUS EFFECTS

The slopes of the dose-response curves for mortality in mice and corneal opacity in guinea pigs are very similar; the serious effect of corneal opacity in guinea pigs occurred at concentrations only a factor of two below the concentrations that caused death in mice. Unfortunately, dose-response data for other nonlethal serious effects are lacking, and there are no quantitative data from humans on serious effects. Thus, it is difficult to predict whether the ERF for corneal opacity in guinea pigs would overestimate or underestimate the risk of effects that could be considered serious in humans. Obviously, exposures should be limited to lower concentrations of HCl to avoid moderate and mild effects.

Data are not available to estimate the incidence of mild or moderate effects in humans or animals. Adequate data are available, however, to estimate a NOEL for mild effects in sensitive humans (i.e., 1.8 ppm for 45 min; see Appendix D), and investigators have identified a possible threshold for mild effects in healthy humans (i.e., 5 ppm for up to 1 hr; see Appendix D). Few data are available to estimate a threshold for moderate effects in healthy adults, and no data are available to estimate a threshold for moderate effects in sensitive individuals. Therefore, the subcommittee examined the possibility of constructing an ERF for mild effects in sensitive humans by using a NOEL for humans as a lower anchor point and the slope of an ERF from animal data. However, the true incidence of mild effects in sensitive humans at the NOEL is unknown. The slope of the ERF could be set equal to the slope of the mortality dose-response in mice (equivalent to the slope of the corneal opacity dose-response in guinea pigs). That construct is based on two assumptions: (1) that the slope of an ERF for humans would be the same as the slope of an ERF for laboratory test animals, and (2) that the slope of an ERF for mild-to-moderate effects would be the same as the slope of an ERF for severe-to-lethal effects. There are problems with both assumptions.

As the heterogenicity of a population increases, a wider range of doses is associated with effects (i.e., the slope of the dose-response curve becomes shallower). Responses to HCl exposure are likely to be more variable in heterogenous human populations downwind of a rocket launch than in a homogenous group of inbred animals. Hence, the slope of an ERF for animals is likely to be more steep than the slope of an ERF for the same end point in a human population. Thus, an ERF based on the slope of an animal dose-response function is likely to overestimate risks to humans if anchored to the human NOEL as a lower bound. This conservative bias, however, might be acceptable to the Air Force.

A more serious problem is the relation between ERFs for mild, moderate, and severe effects. At low exposure concentrations in occupational settings, the irritative effects of HCl appear to be primarily a function of the exposure concentration rather than the concentration multiplied by time (Appendix D). That observation suggests that Haber's law is less applicable as the exposure concentration declines (and the effects become more mild). Thus, it would not be appropriate to plot the incidence of mild effects against cumulative exposure (i.e., $C \times T$) using the same slope as an ERF for severe effects. Instead, it would be necessary to plot the incidence of mild (or moderate) effects as a function of exposure C and T separately, either by multiple regression analysis with two independent variables (C and T) or by plotting separate incidence-versus-concentration ERFs for different exposure durations (e.g., 10, 20, and 30 min). Either approach could be incorporated into the LATRA-ERF model; however, the subcommittee believes that the available toxicological data are insufficient to support either type of model fitting at this time.

NITROGEN DIOXIDE

Available data indicate that exposure to NO_2 can result in a wide variety of respiratory effects in humans and animals (Appendix E). Although the severity of effects increases with increasing exposure concentration and duration, concentration has the more pronounced influence. Reports of exposures at high concentrations for short durations were most often related to accidents, where exposure concentrations were poorly characterized.

Certain groups might be more sensitive to the effects of NO_2 exposure than others; those groups are persons with pre-existing cardiopulmonary problems and children. Lower concentrations of NO_2 might affect those groups more than healthy adults, or the severity of an effect at a given concentration might be greater. The existing data do not clearly indicate a difference in sensitivity among humans to low concentrations of NO_2, and studies have not been conducted on humans using high concentrations. The groups identified above are potentially at risk of more severe reactions than the general population when exposed to very high concentrations of NO_2.

Exposure-response data are available for NO_2 for a number of end points. Of those, the subcommittee attempted to develop ERFs from the most promising data sets: exposure-response data for animal mortality and for human airway responsiveness.

MORTALITY

Hine et al. (1970) exposed rats, mice, guinea pigs, rabbits, and dogs to NO_2 at several concentrations for various durations. In these studies the guinea pig was more susceptible to the lethal effects of NO_2 than the mouse and rat, and the rabbit and dog were relatively more resistant. Reviews of the literature (Mauderly 1984, 1988) indicate that the pulmonary-function responses of the guinea pig to sensory irritants are similar to those observed in humans at low exposure concentrations. Indeed, the guinea pig is used in standard tests for irritancy (Alarie 1973a,b, 1981; Wong and Alarie 1982). However, guinea pigs are more sensitive than other laboratory animals to mortality from exposure to high concentrations of an irritant because the guinea pig's airways tend to completely constrict and occlude the passage of air (Azoulay-Dupuis 1983; EPA 1993). Therefore, the mouse data were used here to construct ERFs. Larsen et al. (1979) considered the mouse to be more sensitive to NO_2 than humans; a mathematical model was used to calculate expected mortality as a function of NO_2 concentrations and exposure durations.

Examination of the mortality data provided by Hine et al. (1970) shows that Haber's rule does not strictly apply for mortality in mice—NO_2 concentration is more important than exposure duration. Using the same type of model adopted by Larsen et al. (1979) for mouse mortality, the standard normal deviate for mortality obtained by a least-squares model fit to the results of Hine et al. (1970) gives

$$z = 3.23 \ln(0.004\ CT^{0.24})$$

where C is concentration in ppm and T is the duration of exposure in minutes. For a mortality risk of 10^{-4} (i.e., the 0.01 percentile), the standard normal deviate is

$$z = -3.72.$$

For an exposure of 5 min, the concentration estimated to produce mortality in 1 in 10,000 mice is obtained from

$$-3.72 = 3.23 \ln(0.004 \times C \times 5^{0.24})$$

giving

$$C = 54 \text{ ppm.}$$

If mice are more sensitive than humans, the risk of death in humans is estimated to be less than 1 in 10,000 for a 5-min exposure to NO_2 at 54 ppm. Similarly, the estimated concentrations for other durations of exposure associated with mortality risks of less than 10^{-4} are shown below.

Duration (min)	HCl (ppm)
5	54
10	45
30	35
60	30

Concentrations estimated for other levels of risk can be obtained by selecting the appropriate value for z. For example, $z = -3.09$ for a risk of 10^{-3} (i.e., the 0.1 percentile of a standard normal distribution).

Gardner et al. (1979) exposed mice to viable microorganisms of *Streptococcus pyogenes* in addition to NO_2 at various concentrations for several durations. For these challenged mice, Larsen et al. (1979) derived a prediction model for the standard normal deviate of

$$z = 1.13 \ln(0.027\, CT^{0.33})$$

where C is the concentration of NO_2 in parts per million and T is the duration of exposure in minutes. At risk levels of 10^{-4}, the mice challenged with *Streptococcus pyogenes* were 70 to 90 times more sensitive for mortality than mice exposed only to NO_2.

AIRWAY RESPONSIVENESS IN HUMANS

Table 15-9 of the U.S. Environmental Protection Agency (EPA 1993) air quality criteria document for NO_2 summarizes the results of several studies investigating airway responses of asthmatic subjects exposed to NO_2 at concentrations of 0.1 to 1.0 ppm for 20 to 120 min. Results were erratic, and airway responsiveness tended to be somewhat less severe in exercising subjects than in resting subjects. Hence, only studies that examined resting subjects were considered here. Airway responsiveness was measured by specific airway conductance or resistance, forced expiratory volume, or total respiratory resistance. Most individuals showed an increase in airway responsiveness, considered a deleterious effect, after NO_2 exposure. However, in some studies, a few individuals showed reduced airway responsiveness. Therefore, the difference in the proportions of individuals showing positive and negative airway responsiveness was used as a measurement of the effect of exposure to NO_2. The subcommittee concluded that the data, listed in Table 6-1, are too erratic to model. The lack of a discernable exposure-response relationship in the data might have been because a small range of concentrations was tested or the experimental conditions varied.

CONTINUOUS (NONQUANTAL) MEASUREMENTS

With quantal (dichotomous) data, risk is defined as the proportion of individuals or animals that are observed to display a specific biological effect (e.g., death, pneumonia, or tearing). Many biological effects do not fall into discrete categories but are measured on a continuous scale (e.g., body weight, breathing rate, or minute volume). For some continuous measurements, an adverse-effect level might have already been established, and risk can be estimated by the proportion of individuals or animals exceeding that level. However, that approach does not make full use of continuous data (Gaylor 1996), and more often than not, an

TABLE 6-1 Airway Responsiveness[a] in Resting Humans with Asthma Exposed to NO_2 (ppm•min < 10)

Number Tested	NO_2, ppm	Duration, min	NO_2 × Duration, ppm•min	Proportion Increased	Proportion Decreased	Proportion Difference
20	0.10	60	6.0	0.65	0.35	0.30
19	0.10	60	6.0	0.53	0.42	0.11
15	0.10	60	6.0	0.40	0.47	- 0.07
20	0.10	60	6.0	0.70	0.15	0.55
7	0.11	60	6.6	—[b]	—[b]	0.00[b]
20	0.14	30	4.2	0.70	0.30	0.40
14	0.25	30	7.5	0.79	0.14	0.65
20	0.27	30	8.1	0.70	0.30	0.40
8	0.48	20	9.6	0.62	0.00	0.62

[a]Data from Table 15-9, EPA (1993) air-quality criteria document for NO_2.
[b]Proportions not listed but authors stated no effect of NO_2.

adverse-effect level for a continuous measurement is not established, particularly for laboratory animals under specific experimental conditions. In such cases, Gaylor and Slikker (1990) developed a technique for estimating risk based on the dose-response relationship and the distribution of measurements (variability among animals) about the dose-response curve. In the absence of a defined adverse-effect level, an "abnormal" level can be defined; for example, the level corresponding to the 1st and 99th percentiles of the unexposed control animals. Then, the probability of animals with abnormal levels can be estimated as a function of dose.

Examples of end points measured on a continuous scale are various measures of pulmonary function in inhalation studies. For example, Januszkiewicz and Mayorga (1994) showed a relationship between lung resistance (R_L), expressed as centimeters of water per liter per second (cmH$_2$O/L-sec), and inhaled exposure dose (D) of NO$_2$, expressed as milligrams per kilogram (mg/kg) of body weight. Sheep were exposed to NO$_2$ at 100 ppm for 15 min or at 500 ppm for 15 to 20 min. Lung resistance was measured 24 hr later. The dose-response relationship from Januszkiewicz and Mayorga (1994) was

$$R_L = 1.3 + 0.72\ D.$$

The measurements in the control animals appear to be adequately described as a normal distribution with a mean of 1.3 and a standard deviation of $s = 0.55$. For this distribution, the 99th percentile was

$$1.3 + (2.33 \times 0.55) = 2.6.$$

Thus, values of lung resistance in sheep above 2.6 cmH$_2$O/L-sec will be considered abnormal. Using that information, it is possible to estimate the risk (probability) of an abnormal level of R_P in sheep as a function of exposure to NO$_2$. For example, suppose one wishes to estimate the exposure at which an additional 10% of the sheep will experience an abnormal level of lung resistance. Because 1% of sheep are by definition in the abnormal range, an excess risk of 10% means the total risk is 11%. Probabilities for normal distributions are calculated from z scores, where z = (measured level − mean)/(standard deviation). The z score corresponding to an upper-tail probability of 0.11 is $z = 1.23$. That is, 11% of the readings exceed 2.6, where

$$z = 1.23 = (2.6 - \text{mean})/0.55,$$

or where the mean = 1.92. Hence,

$$R_L = 1.92 = 1.3 + 0.72\, D$$

and

$$D = 0.86 \text{ mg/kg body weight.}$$

That is, the excess risk of lung resistance in sheep is estimated to be 10% at a dose of NO_2 of 0.86 mg/kg of body weight. Similar calculations for other levels of excess risk are shown in Table 6-2.

If sheep and humans are equally sensitive to NO_2 when expressing dose on the basis of milligrams per kilogram of body weight, then a dose of 0.86 mg/kg corresponding to an excess risk of 10% is 0.86 × 60 = 51.6 mg total of NO_2 for a 60-kg adult. A moderately active human inhales about 1 m³ of air per hour. Thus, in 1 hr, a human inhales 51.6 mg of NO_2 at a concentration of 51.6 mg/m³. Expressed on the basis of milligram minutes per meter cubed, that exposure is equal to 51.6 mg/m³ × 1 hr × 60 min/hr, or 3,096 mg•min/m³ (1,650 ppm•min) for a risk of 10%. Calculations for other levels of excess risk in humans are given in Table 6-3.

Alternatively, suppose the risk of abnormal lung resistance is a function of the air concentration of NO_2 multiplied by the exposure duration instead of a function of the inhaled dose. On the basis of an average minute volume of 7.6 liters (0.0076 m³) in sheep (calculated from measurements reported by Januszkiewicz and Mayorga 1994), an exposure of an average 42-kg sheep to NO_2 at 1 mg/kg body weight, or 42 mg total, is equivalent to an exposure of 42 mg ÷ 0.0076 m³/min = 5,526 mg•min/m³. Hence, an exposure of 0.056 mg/kg is equal to 0.056 × 5,526 = 310 mg•min/m³ or 165 ppm•min for an excess risk of 0.001. Calculations for other levels of excess risk in sheep are given in Table 6-4.

TABLE 6-2 Excess Risk of Increased Lung Resistance (R_L) in Sheep

Excess Risk	Total Risk	z Score	Mean R_L	Exposure (D), mg/kg Body Weight
0.001	0.011	2.29	1.34	0.056
0.01	0.02	2.05	1.47	0.24
0.1	0.11	1.23	1.92	0.86

TABLE 6-3 Excess Risk of Increased Lung Resistance in Humans Based on Data from Sheep

Excess Risk	Exposure			
	mg/kg	mg	mg•min/m^3	ppm•min
0.001	0.056	3.4	204	110
0.01	0.24	14.4	864	460
0.1	0.86	51.6	3096	1650

CONCLUSIONS AND RECOMMENDATIONS

The LATRA model has been developed as an approach for estimating the number of people that might be affected as a result of exposure to toxic emissions from rocket launches. The accuracy of the LATRA predictions depends on the accuracy of the ERFs, which provide an estimate of the incidence of health effects (mild or severe) as a function of exposure. The Air Force procedure for deriving ERFs was described in detail in Chapter 2 and evaluated in Chapter 5.

As described in Chapter 5, the subcommittee recommends using all available and pertinent exposure-response data to establish an ERF via a model-fitting process rather than using only estimates of exposures that might (or might not) correspond to the 1st and 99th percentiles. In this chapter, the subcommittee provided examples for procedures for developing ERFs for HNO_3, HCl, and NO_2. Extensive use was made of Haber's law that predicts effects on the basis of exposure duration times airborne concentrations of chemicals. In some cases, extrapolations across large differences in exposure duration (e.g., from 60 min to 5 min) might result in uncertain predictions. Based on its analysis, the subcommittee concluded that the paucity of exposure-response data for nonlethal end points makes it impossible to construct ERFs for most of the

TABLE 6-4 Excess Risk of Increased Lung Resistance in Sheep

Excess Risk	Exposure			
	mg/kg	mg	mg•min/m^3	ppm•min
	0.056	3.4	310	165
0.01	0.24	14.4	1330	710
0.1	0.86	51.6	4750	2530

situations of interest to the Air Force. However, when an ERF cannot be constructed, it is usually possible to estimate an exposure concentration and duration that is unlikely to result in health effects (i.e., a NOEL). Thus, it should be possible to use LATRA to estimate the number of people who are likely to be exposed at levels exceeding a no-observed-effect level (NOEL) and to indicate the magnitude of the excess (see Chapter 5). That estimate does not provide an estimate of the number of individuals affected or severity of effects, but it does provide an estimate of the number of people at risk from exposures in excess of the NOELs.

For the examples of ERFs constructed in this section, the uncertainty in the measurements of exposure is approximately a factor of two, higher or lower. Hence, estimates of the incidence of effects based on those ERFs would not be accurate. The magnitude of the uncertainty could be determined by calculating the expected number of individuals at risk with the ERFs shifted higher and lower; however, there are additional uncertainties if animal data are used to estimate effects for humans and if the slope of the dose-response relationship for one end point is used to estimate the slope of dose-response relations for another end point.

Given the limited dose-response data available for the rocket-emission toxicants, Chapter 5 recommended that either an expert elicitation process be used to estimate ERFs or the hazard-quotient–hazard-index approach be used to characterize risks. The subcommittee feels that it has exhausted the possibilities for constructing ERFs from incidence data for HCl and HNO_3. The subcommittee did not examine all of the dose-response studies available for NO_2 for their potential to develop ERFs, however. Thus, it is possible that addtional health-end-point-specific ERFs could be developed for NO_2 using one of the approaches described in this chapter and Chapter 5. However, risk characterization will be more clear if the same risk-assessment model is applied to all three rocket-emission toxicants.

REFERENCES

Abraham, W.M., C.S. Kim, M.M. King, W. Oliver, Jr., and L. Yerger. 1982. Effects of HNO_3 on carbochol reactivity of the airways in normal and allergic sheep. Arch. Environ. Health 37:36-40.

Alarie, Y. 1973a. Sensory irritation of the upper airways by airborne chemicals. Toxicol. Appl. Pharmacol. 24:279-297.

Alarie, Y. 1973b. Sensory irritation by airborne chemicals. CRC Crit. Rev. Toxicol. 2:299-363.

Alarie, Y. 1981. Dose-response analysis in animal studies: Prediction of human responses. Environ. Health Perspect. 42:9-13.

Aris, R., D. Christian, I. Tager, L. Ngo, W.E. Finkbeiner, and J.R. Balmes. 1993. Effects of nitric acid gas alone or in combination with ozone on healthy volunteers. Am. Rev. Respir. Dis. 148:965-973.

ATS (American Thoracic Society), Scientific Assembly for Environmental and Occupational Health. 1985. Guidelines as to what constitutes an adverse respiratory health effect, with special reference to epidemiologic studies of air pollution. Am. Rev. Respir. Dis. 131:666-668.

ATS (American Thoracic Society). 1996a. Health effects of outdoor air pollution. Am. J. Respir. Crit. Care Med. 153:3-50.

ATS (American Thoracic Society). 1996b. Health effects of outdoor air pollution. Part 2. Am. J. Respir. Crit. Care Med. 153:477-498.

Azoulay-Dupuis, E., M. Torres, P. Soler, and J. Moreau. 1983. Pulmonary NO_2 toxicity in neonate and adult guinea pigs and rats. Environ. Res. 30:322-339.

Bauer, M.A., M.J. Utell, P.E. Morrow, D.M. Speers, and F.R. Gibb. 1986. Inhalation of 0.30 ppm nitrogen dioxide potentiates exercise-induced bronchospasm in asthmatics. Am. Rev. Respir. Dis. 134:1203-1208.

Berry, M., P.J. Lioy, K. Gelperin, G. Buckler, and J. Klotz. 1991. Accumulated exposure to ozone and measurement of health effects in children and counselors at two summer camps. Environ. Res. 54:135-150.

Brain, J.D., B.D. Beck, J.A. Warren, and R.A. Shaikh, eds. 1988. Variations in Susceptibility to Inhaled Pollutants. Identification, Mechanisms and Policy Implications. Baltimore, Md.: The Johns Hopkins University Press.

Burleigh-Flayer, H., K.L. Wong, and Y. Alarie. 1985. Evaluation of the pulmonary effects of HCl using CO_2 challenges in guinea pigs. Fundam. Appl. Toxicol. 5:978-985.

Calabrese, E.J. 1978. Pollutants and High Risk Groups: The Biological Basis of Increased Human Susceptibility to Environmental and Occupational Pollutants. New York: John Wiley & Sons.

Calabrese, E.J. 1986. Age and Susceptibility to Toxic Substances. New York: John Wiley & Sons.

CDC (Centers for Disease Control and Prevention). 1993. Populations at risk from air pollution—United States. MMWR 42:301-304.

Darmer, K.I., Jr., E.R. Kinkead, and L.C. DiPasquale. 1974. Acute toxicity in rats and mice exposed to hydrogen chloride gas and aerosols. Am. Ind. Hyg. Assoc. J. 35:623-631.

Drew, R.T., G.A. Boorman, J.K. Haseman, E.E. McConnell, W.M. Busey, and J.A. Moore. 1983. The effect of age and exposure duration on cancer induction by a known carcinogen in rats, mice, and hamsters. Toxicol. Appl. Pharmacol. 68:120-130.

Eaton, D.L., and C.D. Klaassen. 1996. Principles of toxicology. Pp. 13-33 in Casarett & Doull's Toxicology: The Basic Science of Poisons, 5th Ed., C.D. Klaassen, M.O. Amdur, and J. Doull, eds. New York: McGraw-Hill.

EPA (U.S. Environmental Protection Agency). 1986. Guidelines for the health risk assessment of chemical mixtures. Fed. Regist. 51(Sept. 24):34014-34025.

EPA (U.S. Environmental Protection Agency). 1989. Risk Assessment Guidance for Superfund, Vol. 1: Human Health. Interim Final. EPA/540/1-89/002. U.S. Environmental Protection Agency, Office of Emergency and Remedial Response, Washington, D.C.

EPA (U.S. Environmental Protection Agency). 1993. Air Quality Criteria for Oxides of Nitrogen, Vol. 3. EPA/600/8-91/049cF. U.S. Environmental Protection Agency, Office of Research and Development, Washington, D.C.

EPA (U.S. Environmental Protection Agency). 1994. Methods for Derivation of Inhalation Reference Concentration and Application of Inhalation Dosimetry. EPA/600/8-90/066F. U.S. Environmental Protection Agency, Office of Research and Development, Washington, D.C.

Evans, J.S., G.M. Gray, R.L. Sielken, Jr., A.E. Smith, C. Valdez-Flores, and J.D. Graham. 1994. Use of probabilistic expert judgment in uncertainty analysis of carcinogenic potency. Regul. Toxicol. Pharmacol. 20(1Pt1):15-36.

Gardner, D.E., F.J. Miller, E.J. Blommer, and D.L. Coffin. 1979. Influence of exposure mode on the toxicity of NO_2. Environ. Health Perspect. 30:23-29.

Gaylor, D.W. 1996. Quantalization of continuous data for benchmark dose estimation. Regul. Toxicol. Pharmacol. 24:246-250.

Gaylor, D.W., and W. Slikker, Jr. 1990. Risk assessment for neurotoxic effects. NeuroToxicology 11:211-218.

Grassman, J.A. 1996. Obtaining information about susceptibility from the epidemiological literature. Toxicology 111:253-270.

Guth, D.J., A.M. Jarabek, L. Wymer, and R.D. Hertzberg. 1991. Evaluation of Risk Assessment Methods for Short-Term Inhalation Exposure. Abstract 91-173.2 in Proceedings of the 84th Annual Meeting of the Air & Waste Management Association. Pittsburgh, Pa.: Air & Waste Management Association.

Hasselblad, V., D.M. Eddy, and D.J. Kotchmar. 1992. Synthesis of environmental evidence: Nitrogen dioxide epidemiology studies. J. Air Waste Manage. Assoc. 42:662-671.

Hertzberg, R.C. and M. Miller. 1985. A statistical model for species extrapolation using categorical response data. Toxicol. Ind. Health 1:43-57.

Hine, C.H., F.H. Meyers, and R.W. Wright. 1970. Pulmonary changes in animals exposed to nitrogen dioxide, effects of acute exposures. Toxicol. Appl. Pharmacol. 16:201-213.

Januszkiewicz, A.J., and M.A. Mayorga. 1994. Nitrogen dioxide induced acute lung injury to sheep. Toxicology 89:279-300.

Klaassen, C.D., M.O. Amdur, and J. Doull, eds. 1996. Casarett & Doull's Toxicology: The Basic Science of Poisons, 5th Ed., New York: McGraw-Hill.

Koenig, J.Q., D.S. Covert, and W.E. Pierson. 1989a. Effects of inhalation of acidic compounds on pulmonary function in allergic adolescent subjects. Environ. Health Perspect. 79:173-178.

Koenig, J.Q., Q.S. Hanley, T.L. Anderson, V. Rebolledo, and W.E. Pierson. 1989b. An Assessment of Pulmonary Function Changes and Oral Ammonia Levels after Exposure of Adolescent Asthmatic Subjects to Sulfuric or Nitric Acid. Abstract 89-92.4 in Proceedings of the 82nd Annual Meeting of the Air & Waste Management Association. Pittsburgh, Pa.: Air & Waste Management Association.

Kovar, M.G., and G.S. Poe. 1985. The National Health Interview Survey design, 1973-84, and procedures, 1975-83. National Center for Health Statistics. Vital Health Stat. Ser. No. 1 (18).

Kreit, J.W., K.B. Gross, T.B. Moore, T.J. Lorenzen, J. D'Arcy, and W.L. Eschenbacher. 1989. Ozone-induced changes in pulmonary function and bronchial responsiveness in asthmatics. J. Appl. Physiol. 66:217-222.

Larsen, R.I., D.E. Gardner, and D.L. Coffin. 1979. An air quality data analysis system for interrelating effects, standards, and needed source reductions: Part 5. NO_2 mortality in mice. J. Air Pollut. Control Assoc. 29:133-137.

Lee, R.C., and W.E. Wright. 1994. Development of human exposure-factor distributions using maximum-entropy inference. J. Exp. Anal. Environ. Epidemiol. 4(3):329-341.

Linn, W.S., D.A. Fischer, D.A. Medway, U.T. Anzar, C.E. Spier, L.M. Valencia, T.G. Venet, and J.D. Hackney. 1982. Short-term respiratory effects of 0.12 ppm ozone exposure in volunteers with chronic obstructive pulmonary disease. Am. Rev. Respir. Dis. 125:658-663.

Linn, W.S., J.C. Solomon, S.C. Trim, C.E. Spier, D.A. Shamoo, T.G. Venet, E.L. Avol, and J.D. Hackney. 1985. Effects of exposure to 4 ppm nitrogen dioxide in healthy and asthmatic volunteers. Arch. Environ. Health 40:234-239.

Linn, W.S., E.L. Avol, R.C. Peng, D.A. Shamoo, and J.D. Hackney. 1987. Replicated dose-response study of sulfur dioxide effects in normal, atopic, and asthmatic volunteers. Am. Rev. Respir. Dis. 136:1127-1134.

Linn, W.S., E.L. Avol, K.R. Anderson, D.A. Shamoo, R.C. Peng, and J.D. Hackney. 1989. Effect of droplet size on respiratory responses to inhaled sulfuric acid in normal and asthmatic volunteers. Am. Rev. Respir. Dis. 140:161-166.

Mattie, D., ed. 1996. Risk Assessment Issues for Sensitive Human Populations. Conference Proceedings, Dayton, Ohio, 25-27 April 1995. Toxicology 111(1-3).

Mauderly, J.L. 1984. Respiratory function responses of animals and man to oxidant gases and to pulmonary emphysema. J. Toxicol. Environ. Health 13:345-361.

Mauderly, J.L. 1988. Comparisons of respiratory functional responses in laboratory animals and man. Pp. 243-261 in The Design and Interpretation of Inhalation Studies and Their Use in Risk Assessment, U. Mohr, ed. New York: Springer-Verlag.

Melia, R.J.W., C. du V. Florey, and S. Chinn. 1979. The relation between respiratory illness in primary schoolchildren and the use of gas for cooking. Results from a national survey. Int. J. Epidemiol. 8:333-338.

Mohsenin, V. 1987. Airway responses to nitrogen dioxide in asthmatic subjects. J. Toxicol. Environ. Health 22:371-380.

Morrow, P.E., and M.J. Utell. 1989. Responses of Susceptible Subpopulations to Nitrogen Dioxide. Res. Rep. 23. Cambridge, Mass.: Health Effects Institute.

Morrow, P.E., M.J. Utell, M.A. Bauer, A.M. Smeglin, M.W. Frampton, C. Cox, D.M. Speers, and F.R. Gibb. 1992. Pulmonary performance of elderly normal subjects and subjects with chronic obstructive pulmonary disease exposed to 0.3 ppm nitrogen dioxide. Am. Rev. Respir. Dis. 145:291-300.

NIOSH (National Institute for Occupational Safety and Health). 1994. Documentation for Immediately Dangerous to Life or Health Concentrations (IDLHs). U.S. Department of Health and Human Services, National Institute for Occupational Safety and Health, Division of Standards Development and Technology Transfer, Cincinnati, Ohio. Available from NTIS, Springfield, Va., Doc. No. PB94-195047.

NRC (National Research Council). 1986. Criteria and Methods for Preparing Emergency Exposure Guidance Level (EEGL), Short-Term Public Emergency Guidance Level (SPEGL), and Continuous Exposure Guidance Level (CEGL) Documents. Washington, D.C.: National Academy Press.

NRC (National Research Council). 1987. Emergency and Continuous Exposure Guidance Levels for Selected Airborne Contaminants. Ammonia, Hydrogen Chloride, Lithium Bromide, and Toluene, Vol. 7. Washington, D.C.: National Academy Press.

NRC (National Research Council). 1988. Complex Mixtures: Methods for In Vivo Toxicity Testing. Washington, D.C.: National Academy Press.

NRC (National Research Council). 1991. Permissible Exposure Levels and Emergency Exposure Guidance Levels for Selected Airborne Contaminants. Washington, D.C.: National Academy Press.

NRC (National Research Council). 1993. Guidelines for Developing Community Emergency Exposure Levels for Hazardous Substances. Washington, D.C.: National Academy Press.

NRC (National Research Council). 1994. Science and Judgment in Risk Assessment. Washington, D.C.: National Academy Press.

NRC (National Research Council). 1997. Toxicity of Military Smokes and Obscurants, Vol. 1. Washington, D.C.: National Academy Press.

Philipson, L.L. 1996. The Exposure-Response Functions of the Launch Area Toxic Risk Analysis (LATRA) Model. Prepared by ACTA Inc., Torrance Calif., and presented to the National Research Council, Committee on Toxicology, at Patrick Air Force Base, Fla. June.

Philipson, L.L., J.M. Hudson, and A.M. See. 1996. Exposure-response functions in Air Force toxic risk modeling. Toxicology 111:239-249.

Poitrast, B.J. 1993. Memorandum to HQ AFSPC/SGB (LTC Martin). Sensitive Populations, A Rule of Thumb. Department of the Air Force, Armstrong Laboratory (AFMC), Brooks Air Force Base, Tex. June.

Seed, J., R.P. Brown, S.S. Olin, and J.A. Foran. 1995. Chemical mixtures: Current risk assessment methodologies and future directions. Regul. Toxicol. Pharmacol. 22:76-94.

Sheppard, D., W.S. Wong, C.F. Uehara, J.A. Nadel, and H.A. Boushey. 1980. Lower threshold and greater bronchomotor responsiveness of asthmatic

subjects to sulfur dioxide. Am. Rev. Respir. Dis. 122:873-878.
Simpson, D.G., R.J. Carroll, H. Zhou, and D.J. Guth. 1996. Interval censoring and marginal analysis in ordinal regression. J. Agric. Biol. Environ. Stat. 1:354-376.
Solic, J.J., M.J. Hazucha, and P.A. Bromberg. 1982. The acute effects of 0.2 ppm ozone in patients with chronic obstructive pulmonary disease. Am. Rev. Respir. Dis. 125:664-669.
Spektor, D.M., M. Lippmann, G.D. Thurston, P.J. Lioy, J. Stecko, G. O'Connor, E. Garshick, F.E. Speizer, and C. Hayes. 1988. Effects of ambient ozone on respiratory function in healthy adults exercising outdoors. Am. Rev. Respir. Dis. 138:821-828.
Spektor, D.M., B.M. Yen, and M. Lippmann. 1989. Effect of concentration and cumulative exposure of inhaled sulfuric acid on tracheobronchial particle clearance in healthy humans. Environ. Health Perspect. 79:167-172.
Stevens, B., J.Q. Koenig, V. Rebolledo, Q.S. Hanley, and D.S. Covert. 1992. Respiratory effects from the inhalation of hydrogen chloride in young adult asthmatics. J. Occup. Med. 34:923-929.
Stokes, M.H. 1994. Memorandum from AL/OEMI to 30 MED Group/SGPB. Consultative Letter, AL/OE-CL-1994=0059, Review of 30 SPW/SEY 12 May 93 Letter to 30 MEDGP/SGPB. Response to AL/OE-CA Consultative Letter, 29 Mar 93.
Turner, D.B. 1994. Workbook of Atmospheric Dispersion Estimates: An Introduction to Dispersion Modeling, 2nd Ed. Boca Raton, Fla.: Lewis.
WHO (World Health Organization). 1992. Acute effects on health of smog episodes. WHO Regional Publications, European Series No. 43. Geneva: World Health Organization.
Wohlslagel, J., L. DiPasquale, and E. Vernot. 1976. Toxicity of solid rocket motor exhaust: Effects of HCl, HF, and alumina on rodents. J. Combust. Toxicol. 3:61-69.
Wong, K.L., and Alarie, Y. 1982. A method for repeated evaluation of pulmonary performance in unanesthetized, unrestrained guinea pigs and its application to detect effects of sulfuric acid mist inhalation. Toxicol. Appl. Pharmacol. 63:72-90.

Appendix A

AIR FORCE EXPOSURE LIMITS FOR ROCKET EMISSIONS

This appendix provides additional background information on three topics: (1) the nature of the rocket emissions; (2) the Air Force's tier limit system of acceptable human exposure criteria for three of those emissions—hydrogen chloride (HCl), nitrogen tetroxide (N_2O_4)-dioxide (NO_2), and nitric acid (HNO_3); and (3) the relationship of the tier limits to the toxicity reference values used to quantify the Launch Area Toxic Risk Analysis (LATRA) exposure-response functions (ERFs).

ROCKET EMISSIONS

The Air Force needs to evaluate risks to human health from rocket emissions at two locations: Vandenberg Air Force Base (VAFB), Western Range, and the Cape Canaveral Air Station (CCAS), Eastern Range. The intercontinental ballistic missile (ICBM) test program (including the Minuteman III and Peacekeeper) and the polar orbit space launches are carried out at Vandenberg; the equatorial and low inclination launches and shuttle-mission support occur at Cape Canaveral. The rockets and missiles launched at both ranges are powered by motors using specified solid or liquid propellants or both. The potentially toxic emissions resulting from these propellants are HCl, NO_2, HNO_3, hydrazines, and lesser amounts of other substances.

HCl is emitted from rockets using solid-propellant motors, usually the first stage of a launch vehicle, and the nitrogen-based compounds are emitted from rockets using liquid propellants, a first or later stage of a launch vehicle. Solid-propellant motors burn a hydrocarbon fuel with ammonium perchlorate as the oxidizer. The resulting rocket emissions at ground level include other combustion products (e.g., CO, CO_2, N_2, H_2, and H_2O) as well as HCl, but the Air Force has considered HCl to be the most hazardous. Liquid-propellant motors often use Aerozine-50 (50:50 blend of hydrazine and unsymmetrical dimethyl hydrazine) as the fuel and N_2O_4 as the oxidizer. For normal launches, nitrogen oxide emissions at ground level are negligible. However, in the case of an accident during fuel transfer or a catastrophic abort near the ground, large quantities of N_2O_4 can be released. In the atmosphere, some of the N_2O_4 is rapidly converted to NO_2. The Air Force speculates that NO_2 rapidly converts further to HNO_3 (T. Clapp, U.S. Air Force Space Command, personal commun., February 25, 1997).

Aerozine-50 also can be released from rockets using liquid propellants in catastrophic aborts (or during transfer operations); however, the Air Force did not ask the subcommittee to review the toxicity of hydrazines for this report. COT recently reviewed the toxicity of hydrazine for the National Aeronautics and Space Administration (NASA) (NRC 1996).

The Air Force has measured and estimated rocket-emission exposure concentrations and durations in the event of normal and catastrophic launches. Projected exposure concentrations and durations during a normal Titan IV launch and a catastrophic abort at Vandenberg are listed below (D. Dargitz, U.S. Air Force 30th Space Wing; L. Philipson, ACTA Inc.; and T. Clapp, U.S. Air Force Space Command; personal commun., March 14, 1997):

A. Normal launch
Peak HCl concentration reaches $\approx$30 parts per million (ppm) out to 3 kilometers (km) downwind
   Range of passage times
      $\geq$10 ppm, $\approx$2 min (7 km)
      $\geq$5 ppm, $\approx$3 min (15 km)
      $\geq$2 ppm, $\approx$4 min (15 km)

B. Catastrophic launch abort
   1. Peak HCl concentration reaches $\approx$90 ppm out to 4 km for an abort 20 sec after takeoff

Range of passage times
≥10 ppm, ≈10 min (5 km)
≥5 ppm, ≈12 min (36 km)
≥2 ppm, ≈16 min (36 km)

2. Peak NO_2 concentration reaches ≈50 ppm out to 7 km
Range of passage times
≥10 ppm, ≈3 min (8 km)
≥4 ppm, ≈4 min (27 km)

Similar short passage times are expected for the ground clouds emanating from the other types of vehicles (e.g., Delta and Atlas rockets, Minuteman and Peacekeeper missiles, and the space shuttle) launched at the Eastern and Western Ranges.

DEFINITIONS OF TIER LIMITS

As noted in Chapter 1, the Air Force initially developed acceptable human exposure levels for the rocket-emission toxicants for military and civilian populations called tier limits. The toxicity information supporting the tier limits influenced the selection of exposure concentrations associated with 1% and 99% incidence of effect in sensitive and normal populations included in LATRA ERFs, as noted in Table 2-1. Derivation of the tier limit values is described below.

The Air Force adopted a three-tiered concept to delineate acceptable exposure concentrations and durations for the public (tier 1), government and contractor personnel on the ranges (tier 2), and operational personnel directly involved with the launch (tier 3). The concept is similar to the three-tier system proposed for the emergency response planning guidelines (ERPGs) of EPA (1987; see box) and comparable to a system proposed by the California Environmental Protection Agency to meet the requirements of the California air toxics "hot spots" law (Cal EPA 1995).

The Air Force defines the tier 1 exposure limit (the outermost tier) as the airborne exposure concentration that poses no hazard to the general population but might affect certain sensitive individuals (e.g., individuals with asthma or emphysema and people with certain other lung

> **EMERGENCY RESPONSE PLANNING GUIDELINES**
>
> **ERPG-3:** The maximum airborne concentration below which it is believed that nearly all individuals could be exposed for up to 1 hr without experiencing or developing life-threatening health effects.
>
> **ERPG-2:** The maximum airborne concentration below which it is believed that nearly all individuals could be exposed for up to 1 hr without experiencing or developing irreversible or other serious health effects or symptoms that could impair an individual's ability to take protective action.
>
> **ERPG-1:** The maximum airborne concentration below which it is believed that nearly all individuals could be exposed for up to 1 hr without experiencing other than mild, transient adverse health effects or perceiving a clearly defined objectionable odor.
>
> Adapted from Organization Resources Counselors (1987) as cited by EPA (1987)

diseases; U.S. Air Force 1997).[1] If tier 1 concentrations are exceeded beyond the base, the Air Force notifies public officials.

The Air Force defines the tier 2 exposure limit (the middle tier) as the airborne exposure concentration that might cause short-term symptoms that most individuals could endure without experiencing or developing irreversible or other serious health effects or symptoms that could impair their ability to take protective action. For personnel in areas with a tier 2 concentration, the Air Force recommends seeking shelter and evacuation (Killan 1994). If tier 2 concentrations are predicted to overlay unprotected population centers (e.g., a single house, building, or facility

---

[1] There are differences between the Eastern and Western Range interpretations of the tier limits; the definitions provided here were developed by the Western Range. (For the Eastern Range tier limits, see Toxic Hazard Control, Daily and Launch Operations (U.S. Air Force 45th Space Wing, 1998)). Although the types of effects in sensitive individuals were not defined in the documentation provided to the subcommittee, the subcommittee assumes that the effects would be as described for ERPG-1.

or, in the case of residential or commercial areas, a small area encompassing houses, stores, etc.) on- or off-base, the Air Force wing safety office recommends a launch hold to the wing commander.

The Air Force defines the tier 3 exposure limit (the innermost tier surrounding the launch pad) as an airborne exposure concentration that can be immediately dangerous to life and health (IDLH). Tier 3 exposure concentrations are based on the NIOSH IDLH (1994) values (U.S. Air Force 1997). Areas within tier 3 concentrations warrant immediate isolation and evacuation actions to prevent exposure (Poitrast 1993; Killan 1994).

Definitions of IDLH and other short-term exposure limits established by various groups and referred to in this report are provided in Appendix B.

In 1994, the Air Force Space Command Surgeon General established the Rocket Emissions Working Group (REWG) to review and provide recommendations for the three-tier limits for HCl and N_2O_4 (NO_2). REWG consisted of personnel from the Air Force Armstrong Laboratory, the U.S. Environmental Protection Agency (EPA), the Lawrence Livermore Laboratory, ACTA, Inc., and others. The Air Force has changed some of the tier limit values on the basis of recommendations from REWG; REWG-recommended tier limits for rocket-emission toxicants are listed in Table A-1.

The Rocket Exhaust Effluent Diffusion Model (REEDM) output is used to identify the locations encompassed by a ground plume concentration exceeding each tier limit, and actions and decisions on whether to launch are made on the basis of the tier-concentration contours relative to the populations defined for each tier (Poitrast 1993).[2]

---

[2]REEDM and LATRA are used somewhat differently at the Eastern and Western Ranges. VAFB operates LATRA, which contains a subset of REEDM, as the single toxic-risk-analysis model used as a basis for go/no-go recommendations to the wing commander. At CCAS, REEDM is used in a stand-alone configuration for go/no-go recommendations; LATRA is operated before the launch to help determine the levels of risk to which off-base population centers can be exposed (D. Dargitz, U.S. Air Force 30th Space Wing, personal commun., March 14, 1997).

TABLE A-1 REWG Recommendations for Air Force Tier Exposure Limits for Rocket-Emission Toxicants

	Tier 3 (inner), ppm	Tier 2 (middle), ppm	Tier 1 (outer), ppm
HCl	50, ceiling (IDLH)	10, ceiling	2, 1-hr TWA (2 × SPEGL); 10, ceiling
N_2O_4 (as NO_2)	20, 30-min TWA (IDLH)	2, 1-hr TWA (IDLH/10); 4, ceiling	0.2, 1-hr TWA; 2, ceiling
HNO_3	25, 30-min TWA (IDLH)	2.5, 1-hr TWA (IDLH/10); 4, ceiling; or 0.3-1.0, 1-hr TWA[a]	0.3, ceiling; or 0.025, 1-hr TWA; 0.05, ceiling[a]

[a] Revisions suggested by Jeffrey I. Daniels, Lawrence Livermore National Laboratory, personal commun., to John Hinz, Armstrong Laboratory, October 25, 1995.

Abbreviations: IDLH, immediately dangerous to life and health; TWA, time-weighted average; SPEGL short-term public emergency guidance levels.

COMPARISON OF REWG TIER RECOMMENDATIONS AND LATRA ERFS

The Air Force used REWG's recommended tier limits to adjust the toxicity values initially used to quantify the LATRA ERFs (see Philipson et al. 1996). REWG tier 1 recommendations, chosen to protect the more sensitive members of the general population, correspond to the 1% effect level (or lower) for adverse effects in sensitive populations in LATRA. The definition of REWG tier 2 corresponds less directly to the LATRA-ERF structure, but was used to set the 1% incidence levels of the LATRA ERFs for normal individuals. REWG considered that the individuals most likely to be exposed to tier 2 concentrations would be the on-base community of military personnel, workers involved in base operations, and their dependents living on base. Although those individuals usually represent a younger and healthier portion of the general population, they might still contain some percentage of sensitive responders. The tier 2 exposure limit might cause some workers to seek medical attention. At one time, tier 3 limits were considered for setting the 99% effect level for ERFs for serious effects in sensitive individuals, but a 5-fold multiple of the 1% effect concentration was selected instead (see Chapter 2).

REFERENCES

Cal EPA (California Environmental Protection Agency). 1995. Technical Support Document for the Determination of Acute Toxicity Exposure Levels for Airborne Toxicants. Draft for Public Comment. Office of Environmental Health Hazard Assessment, Sacramento, Calif. January.

EPA (U.S. Environmental Protection Agency). 1987. Technical Guidance for Hazards Analysis: Emergency Planning for Extremely Hazardous Substances. Prepared in cooperation with the Federal Emergency Management Agency, Washington, D.C., and U.S. Department of Transportation, Washington, D.C. U.S. Environmental Protection Agency, Office of Solid Waste and Emergency Response, Washington, D.C. Available from NTIS, Springfield, Va., Doc. No. PB93-206910.

Killan, G.A. 1994. Memorandum from HQ AFSPC/SECE to meeting attendees. Toxic Risk Analysis Models and Exposure Limits Meeting Minutes. U.S. Air Force Space Command.

NIOSH (National Institute for Occupational Safety and Health). 1994. Documentation for Immediately Dangerous to Life or Health Concentrations (IDLHs). U.S. Department of Health and Human Services, National Institute for Occupational Safety and Health, Division of Standards Development and Technology Transfer, Cincinnati, Ohio. Available from NTIS, Springfield, Va., Doc. No. PB94-195047.

NRC (National Research Council). 1986. Criteria and Methods for Preparing Emergency Exposure Guidance Level (EEGL), Short-Term Public Emergency Guidance Level (SPEGL), and Continuous Exposure Guidance Level (CEGL) Documents. Washington, D.C.: National Academy Press.

NRC (National Research Council). 1996. Spacecraft Maximum Allowable Concentrations for Selected Airborne Contaminants, Vol. 2. Washington, D.C., National Academy Press.

Organization Resources Counselors. 1987. Memorandum to ORC Occupational Safety and Health Group from Darrell K. Mattheis and Rebecca L. Daiss, update on Emergency Response Planning Guidelines (ERPG) Task Force. Organization Resources Counselors, Washington, D.C. July 20, 1987.

Philipson, L.L., J.M. Hudson, and A.M. See. 1996. Exposure-response functions in Air Force toxic risk modeling. Toxicology 111:239-249.

Poitrast, B.J. 1993. Memorandum to HQ AFSPACECOM/SGPB 30 MEDGP/SGPB. Consultative letter, AL-CL-1993-0058, Evaluation of Three-Tier Exposure Philosophy and Tier Limits, Vandenberg AFB Calif. Department of the Air Force, Armstrong Laboratory (AFMC), Brooks Air Force Base, Tex. March.

U.S. Air Force 30th Space Wing. 1997. Toxic Hazard Assessments. 30th Space

Wing Instruction 91-106. 30th Space Wing, Air Force Space Command Range Safety Office, Vandenberg Air Force Base, Calif.

U.S. Air Force 45th Space Wing. 1998. Toxic Hazard Control, Daily and Launch Operations. 45th Space Wing Range Safety Operations Requirement No. 19, 24 March 1998. Patrick Air Force Base, Fla.

Appendix B

DEFINITIONS OF CURRRENT EXPOSURE GUIDANCE LEVELS

Emergency Response Planning Guidelines (ERPGs) are developed by the American Industrial Hygiene Association. Definitions of ERPG-1 (mild effects), ERPG-2 (serious effects), and ERPG-3 (life-threatening effects) are provided in the box in Chapter 1. ERPGs are intended to protect "nearly all individuals" from each effect level. In establishing ERPGs, acute toxicity data as well as possible long-term effects from a single acute exposure are considered. Adjustments, based on informed judgment, can be made for the increase susceptibility of sensitive subgroups in the general population (EPA 1987, Appendix D).

Immediately Dangerous to Life and Health (IDLH) values are used by the National Institute for Occupational Safety and Health (NIOSH) as respirator selection criteria (first developed in the mid-1970s). The Occupational Safety and Health Administration (OSHA) defines an IDLH as: "An atmospheric concentration of any toxic, corrosive or asphyxiant substance that poses an immediate threat to life or would cause irreversible or delayed adverse health effects or would interfere with an individual's ability to escape from a dangerous atmosphere" (29 CFR 1910.120).

A joint effort was called the Standards Completion Program (SCP), whereby NIOSH and OSHA cooperated to develop draft standards (NIOSH 1978). The definition of an IDLH that was developed during the SCP considered the ability of a worker to escape a building. Although egress from a particular worksite could occur in much less than 30 min in most cases, as a margin of safety, IDLHs were based on effects

Appendix B: Definitions of Exposure Guidance Levels

that might occur as a consequence of a 30-min exposure (NIOSH 1994).

The criteria used to determine the adequacy of existing IDLHs were a combination of those used during the SCP and a new method developed by NIOSH (tiered data preference). Acute lethal animal data could be used but would be time adjusted to a 30-min exposure period according to the formula:

$$\text{Adjusted LC}_{50} \text{ (30 min)} = \text{LC}_{50}(t) \times (t/0.5)^{1/n}$$

where $\text{LC}_{50}(t)$ is an LC_{50} determined over t hours and n is a constant determined empirically (NIOSH 1994).

EPA Levels of Concern (LOC) are the "concentrations of an extremely hazardous substance (EHS) in air above which there may be serious irreversible health effects or death as a result of a single exposure for a relatively short period of time" (EPA 1987). For purposes of the December 1987 *Technical Guidance for Hazard Analysis, Emergency Planning for Extremely Hazardous Substances*, EPA defined LOCs as 1/10 of NIOSH IDLH levels.

Emergency Exposure Guidance Levels (EEGLs) are concentrations of substances in the air that may be judged by the U.S. Department of Defense to be acceptable for the performance of specific tasks during rare, emergency conditions, lasting 1 to 24 hr (NRC 1986). The EEGL should allow personnel to continue to perform tasks necessary to take care of the emergency conditions and to allow self-rescue. Therefore, the EEGL should not impair judgment, interfere with performance of tasks in response to the emergency, or cause irreversible harm to the personnel. The EEGL may, however, cause transient adverse effects, such as increased respiration rate, headache (but not debilitating headache), mild central-nervous-system effects, or irritation to the eyes or upper respiratory tract. An EEGL is acceptable only during an emergency, when some discomfort or risk must be taken to avoid greater risks, such as fire, explosion, or massive releases of toxic material (NRC 1986).

The calculation of an EEGL is based on the exposure population being military personnel who are healthy and relatively young. Women are included; thus, the potential toxicity of the exposure material to the fetus is considered. Personnel are expected to have appropriate protective equipment available and to have planned escape routes, but EEGLs are not based on the availability of the protective equipment or escape routes (NRC 1986).

Short-Term Public Emergency Guidance Levels (SPEGLs) are suitable concentrations for single, short-term, emergency exposures of the general public (NRC 1986). SPEGLs are developed at the request of the U.S. Department of Defense for emergency situations in which the public might be involved. Sensitive populations, such as children, the aged, and persons with serious, debilitating diseases (NRC 1986), are considered in SPEGLs.

Acute Exposure Guideline Levels (AEGLs) are under development by the U.S. Army and U.S. Environmental Protection Agency. There are likely to be three levels of AEGL: Below AEGL-1, exposure levels might produce mild odor, taste, or other mild sensory irritations in the general population, including sensitive individuals. Below AEGL-2 but above AEGL-1, exposure levels might cause notable discomfort in the general population. Below AEGL-3 but above AEGL-2, exposure levels might cause irreversible or other serious long-lasting effects or impaired ability to escape. Above AEGL-3, exposure levels might cause life-threatening effects or death in the general population, including sensitive individuals. The AEGL definitions might not be final.

ACGIH Threshold Limit Values (TLVs) are based on available information from industrial experience, from experimental human and animal studies, and when possible, from a combination of the three. The basis on which the values are established might differ from substance to substance; protection against impairment of health might be a guiding factor for some values, whereas reasonable freedom from irritation, narcosis, nuisances, or other forms of stress might be the basis for others. Health impairments under consideration are those that shorten life expectancy, compromise physiological function, impair the capability to resist other toxic substances of disease processes, or adversely affect reproductive function or developmental processes (ACGIH 1986).

ACGIH TLV Time-Weighted Averages (TWAs) are defined as time-weighted-average concentration limits for a normal 8-hr workday, with a total of 40 hr per week. Nearly all workers can be exposed repeatedly, day after day, to these concentrations without adverse effects (ACGIH 1986).

ACGIH TLV Short-Term Exposure Limits (STELs) are 15-min time-weighted-average concentrations for a normal 8-hr workday and 40-hr workweek. All workers should be able to withstand up to four exposures per day of concentrations as high as the TLV-STEL with no ill effects if the TLV-TWA is not exceeded. TLV-STELs are applied to supplement the TLV-TWA when there are recognized acute effects from a substance whose toxic effects are primarily chronic in nature (ACGIH 1986).

ACGIH TLV Ceiling (C) limits are airborne concentrations that should not be exceeded in the workplace under any circumstances. Ceiling limits can supplement other limits or stand alone. For chemicals with TLV-TWA values for which ACGIH could not find sufficent toxicity data to derive TLV-STELs or TLV-C values, ACGIH recommends that five times the TLV-TWA be used in place of the TLV-C and that only three short-term exposures to that level for up to 30 min per day be allowed (ACGIH 1986).

OSHA Permissible Exposure Limits (PELs) are workplace exposure standards listed in the General Industry Standards for Toxic and Hazardous Chemicals (29 CFR 1910, Subpart Z). Most of the PELs are based on ACGIH TLVs. PELs for many chemicals are simply 8-hr time-weighted-average (TWA) concentrations that should not be exceeded in an 8-hr workday. For other chemicals, ceiling concentrations and maximum peak concentrations are given in addition to the 8-hr TWA concentrations. The maximum peak concentrations apply to specific exposure durations (e.g., 5-min maximum peak concentrations in any 2-hr period). The concentrations should never exceed the maximum peak and should fall between the ceiling and the maximum peak concentrations for the duration indicated. The majority of OSHA PELs were adopted from the ACGIH TLVs available in 1971. PELs are enforceable by law (EPA 1987).

NIOSH Recommended Exposure Limits (RELs) are 8-hr or 10-hr TWA or ceiling concentrations (EPA 1987).

REFERENCES

ACGIH (American Conference of Governmental Industrial Hygienists). 1986. Threshold Limit Values and Biological Exposure Indices for 1986-87. American Conference of Governmental Industrial Hygienists, Cincinnati, Ohio.

EPA (U.S. Environmental Protection Agency). 1987. Technical Guidance for Hazards Analysis: Emergency Planning for Extremely Hazardous Substances. Prepared in cooperation with the Federal Emergency Management Agency, Washington, D.C., and U.S. Department of Transportation, Washington, D.C. U.S. Environmental Protection Agency, Office of Solid Waste and Emergency Response, Washington, D.C. Available from NTIS, Springfield, Va., Doc. No. PB93-206910.

NIOSH (National Institute for Occupational Safety and Health). 1978. The Standards Completion Program Draft Technical Standards Analysis and Decision Logics. U.S. Department of Health and Human Services, National Institute for Occupational Safety and Health, Cincinnati, Ohio.

NIOSH (National Institute for Occupational Safety and Health). 1994. Documentation for Immediately Dangerous to Life or Health Concentrations (IDLHs). U.S. Department of Health and Human Services, National Institute for Occupational Safety and Health, Division of Standards Development and Technology Transfer, Cincinnati, Ohio. Available from NTIS, Springfield, Va., Doc. No. PB94-195047.

NRC (National Research Council). 1986. Criteria and Methods for Preparing Emergency Exposure Guidance Level (EEGL), Short-Term Public Emergency Guidance Level (SPEGL), and Continuous Exposure Guidance Level (CEGL) Documents. Washington, D.C.: National Academy Press.

Appendix C

AMERICAN THORACIC SOCIETY'S LIST OF ADVERSE RESPIRATORY HEALTH EFFECTS

THE American Thoracic Society's Scientific Assembly for Environmental and Occupational Health list of adverse respiratory effects is presented below in order from most to least severe.

A. Increased mortality. (Increased as used here and subsequently means significantly ($p < 0.05$) increased above that recorded in some standard, comparable population. In selected situations, $p < 0.1$ might be appropriate.)
B. Increased incidence of cancer.
C. Increased frequency of symptomatic asthmatic attacks.
D. Increased incidence of lower respiratory tract infections.
E. Increased exacerbations of disease in persons with chronic cardiopulmonary or other disease that could be reflected in a variety of ways:
    1. Less able to cope with daily activities (e.g. shortness of breath or increased anginal episodes).
    2. Increased hospitalizations, both frequency and duration.
    3. Increased emergency ward or physician visits.
    4. Increased pulmonary medication.
    5. Decreased pulmonary function.
F. Reduction in forced expiratory volume (FEV), or forced vital capacity (FVC) or other tests of pulmonary function:
    1. Chronic reduction in FEV or FVC associated with clinical symptoms.

2. A significant increase in number of persons with FEV below normal limits: chronically reduced FEV is a predictor of increased risk of mortality. Transient or reversible reductions that are not associated with an asthmatic attack appear to be less important. It should be emphasized that a small, but statistically significant, reduction in a population mean FEV, or $FEV_{0.75}$, is probably medically significant, because such a difference may indicate an increase in the number of persons with respiratory impairment in the population. In other words, a small part of the population may manifest a marked change that is medically significant to them, but when averaged with the rest of the population, the change appears to be small.
3. An increased rate of decline in pulmonary function (FEV_1) relative to predicted value in adults with increasing age or failure of children to maintain their predicted FEV_1 growth curve. Such data must be standardized for sex, race, height, and other demographic and anthropometric factors.

G. Increased prevalence of wheezing in the chest apart from colds, or of wheezing most days or nights. (The significance of wheezing with colds needs more study and evaluation.)
H. Increased prevalence or incidence of chest tightness.
I. Increased prevalence or incidence of cough/phlegm production requiring medical attention.
J. Increased incidence of acute upper respiratory tract infections that interfere with normal activity.
K. Acute upper respiratory tract infections that do not interfere with normal activity.
L. Eye, nose, and throat irritation that might interfere with normal activity (i.e., driving a car) if severe.

REFERENCES

ATS (American Thoracic Society), Scientific Assembly for Environmental and Occupational Health. 1985. Guidelines as to what constitutes an adverse respiratory health effect, with special reference to epidemiologic studies of air pollution. Am. Rev. Respir. Dis. 131:666-668.

Appendix D

ACUTE TOXICITY OF HYDROGEN CHLORIDE

BACKGROUND INFORMATION

HYDROGEN chloride (HCl) is a colorless, corrosive gas with a pungent, suffocating odor. It is highly soluble in water, forming hydrochloric acid. HCl can occur in gaseous and aerosol forms in the atmosphere, and its partitioning between the two is dependent on temperature and humidity (Sebacher et al. 1980). Lower ambient temperature and higher relative humidity in the atmosphere favor aerosol formation (Sebacher et al. 1980). The gas-liquid equilibrium is also affected by available droplet nucleation sites, which are plentiful in rocket-exhaust clouds. Inhaled HCl in contact with moisture in the upper respiratory tract is expected to rapidly disassociate because of its high water solubility.

PHYSICAL AND CHEMICAL PROPERTIES

CAS No.:	7647-01-0
Molecular formula:	HCl
Molecular weight:	36.47
Chemical name:	Hydrogen chloride
Synonyms:	Muriatic acid, spirits of salt, chlorohydric acid, hydrochloric acid gas
Physical state:	Gas
Boiling point:	-84.9°C
Melting point:	-144.8°C

Vapor density: 1.26 (air = 1.0)
Vapor pressure: 40 mm Hg at 17.8°C
Solubility: Highly soluble in water, forming hydrochloric acid (82.3 g/100 g of water at 0°C)
Color: Colorless as a gas
Conversion factors at 25°C, 1 atm: 1 ppm = 1.49 mg/m^3
1 mg/m^3 = 0.671 ppm

Sources and Occurrence

HCl can be produced by several methods. The majority (90%) of the HCl produced in the United States is a by-product of various chlorination processes (Hisham and Bommaraju 1995). Lesser amounts (8%) are produced directly from hydrogen (H_2) and chlorine (Cl_2). Combustion of chlorine-containing organic compounds results in the formation of HCl. Average HCl concentrations in combustion flue gas have been reported as high as 3,030 ppm (Sebacher et al. 1980). HCl is also found naturally in volcanic gases particularly in Mexico and South America and might have been one of the gases in the original atmosphere of the earth (Hisham and Bommaraju 1995). HCl from sea salt is the main source of tropospheric HCl from natural sources (Symonds et al. 1988). Combustion of fossil fuels (especially coal) is the most common anthropogenic source of ambient HCl concentrations, which have been measured in the range of 0.5-7.6 ppb (Kamrin 1992). In areas near sources of HCl from combustion, Kamrin (1992) estimated the maximum HCl concentrations to be in the range of 20-30 ppb.

HCl is formed during the combustion of rocket propellants containing ammonium perchlorate (NH_4ClO_4). The major combustion reaction producing HCl is

$$C_nH_m + NH_4ClO_4 \rightarrow CO + CO_2 + HCl + N_2 + H_2 + H_2O.$$

The HCl concentration in the exit plane of a solid propellant rocket using ammonium perchlorate as an oxidizer was calculated to be 18.31-19.41 grams (g)/100 g of propellant burned for three types of rockets (Bennett 1996). Pellett et al. (1983) reported that the exhaust from a space-shuttle launch using a solid rocket fuel contained 60 tons of HCl. The total range of peak HCl concentrations measured in eight Titan III rocket altitude-stabilized exhaust clouds was 25-0.5 ppm (for 3-300 min) (Pellett et al. 1983). Partitioning studies indicated that total hydrochloric acid produced by a U.S. space-shuttle launch was predominantly an aerosol, but due to the rapid dissipation of the aerosol, the gas phase was the predominant state within several minutes of the launch (Sebacher et al. 1980). At equilibrium under unpolluted tropospheric concentrations of HCl (less than 1 ppb), the gas phase will predominate except at high (more than 90%) humidity (Sebacher et al. 1980).

PHARMACOKINETICS AND METABOLISM

Due to its high solubility, HCl rapidly forms hydrochloric acid when it comes in contact with water. HCl dissociates in water to form hydronium ions (H_3O^+) that can interact with tissue elements, resulting in cell injury or death (Perry et al. 1994). The predominant effects of inhaled HCl are due to local tissue contact, particularly in the upper respiratory tract. Due to the high reactivity of HCl with the upper respiratory tract, significant systemic exposure to HCl is unlikely. Absorption of substantial amounts of inhaled HCl might decrease blood pH; however, such an effect has not been observed even at high exposure concentrations. Kaplan et al. (1988) exposed baboons to HCl at 500, 5,000, or 10,000 ppm and measured blood pH. Blood pH was transiently reduced at the highest exposure concentration, but the differences were not statistically significant and were most likely due to alterations in blood gas levels. Ammonia in exhaled air increased in men and women volunteers who inhaled HCl at 0.8 or 1.8 ppm (Stevens et al. 1992). The increase in ammonia might indicate a mechanism for neutralization of HCl in the upper airways.

Pharmacokinetic studies with HCl have not been conducted, but hydrogen and chloride ions are involved in normal physiological processes. Hydrochloric acid is an important normal constituent of gastric juice. Humans ingesting 50 millimoles (mmol) per day of hydrochloric acid for 4 days had reduced blood and urinary urea and an increase in excretion of ammonia (Fine et al. 1977). Intravenous infusion of 0.15 molarity hydrochloric acid into rats (50 milliliters per kilogram (mL/kg) of body weight per hour) and dogs (20 mL/kg of body weight per hour) increased urinary chloride excretion (Kotchen et al. 1980).

SUMMARY OF TOXICITY INFORMATION

EFFECTS IN HUMANS

One-Time Exposure

The National Research Council reviewed the toxicological effects of HCl in humans (NRC 1987, 1991). The reports concluded that exposure to irritating concentrations of HCl can result in coughing, pain, inflammation, edema, and desquamation in the upper respiratory tract. Acute exposure to high concentrations might produce constriction of the larynx and bronchi and closure of the glottis. Because HCl is highly irritating to the mucosal surfaces of the respiratory tract and the eyes, it has good warning properties.

Henderson and Haggard (1943) summarized information from several sources related to how long various exposure concentrations of HCl could be tolerated by healthy workers and what effects might occur (Table D-1). Matt (1889) stated in his doctoral dissertation that work is impossible when one inhales air containing HCl in concentrations of 50 to 100 ppm; work is difficult but possible when the air contains concentrations of 10 to 50 ppm; and work is undisturbed at the concentration of 10 ppm. However, the exposure protocol used by Matt (1889) included only two individuals and three exposure concentrations. Each individual was exposed once to HCl at 10 ppm (10 min), 70 ppm (15 min), and 100 ppm (15 min). When exposed at 70 ppm, the individuals left the exposure chamber once briefly during the 15-min period, and when exposed at 100 ppm, they left several times because of their acute discomfort. During exposure at the high concentrations, the individuals experienced coughing, increased breathing frequency, and strong irritation of the throat and respiratory tract. Matt (1889) included in his report a description by another investigator of an additional volunteer exposed to HCl at 50 ppm for 13 min. Heyroth (1963) indicated in an editorial note that it was his opinion that most people can detect HCl in the air at 1-5 ppm and that 5-10 ppm is a disagreeable exposure concentration. Elkins (1959) was of the opinion that exposure to HCl at 5 ppm is immediately irritating to the nose and throat, but without long lasting effects. Sayers et al. (1934) expressed an opinion that prolonged exposure to 1-5 ppm resulted in slight symptoms, exposure to 5-10 ppm for 1 hr was the maximum exposure concentration without serious effects, and 150-200 ppm was dangerous in 30-60 min.

TABLE D-1 Interpretations of Various HCl Exposure Concentrations in the Workplace

HCl Concentration, ppm	Exposure Duration	Physiological Responses	References
1,000-2,000	Brief	Dangerous for even short exposures	Henderson and Haggard 1943
50-100	1 hr	Maximum tolerable concentration	Henderson and Haggard 1943
10-50	A few hr	Maximum tolerable concentration	Henderson and Haggard 1943
35	Unspecified short time	Irritation of throat	Henderson and Haggard 1943
10	Prolonged	Maximum allowable concentration	Henderson and Haggard 1943
1-5	—	Odor threshold	Heyroth 1963

Accidental Exposures

One report described a spill of approximately 380,000 L of HCl onto the ground from a storage tank containing 32% HCl in solution. Fire fighters in protective equipment controlled the spill; however, several of the response personnel developed facial rashes 2-3 days later. The HCl exposure responsible for the rashes was due to shifting winds, which increased the acid exposure to the faces of the responders (Hazardous Substances Data Bank 1996).

A clinical study involving 170 fire fighters identified HCl from degradation of polyvinyl chloride as an important contributor to respiratory symptoms. One death with hemorrhage, edema, and inflammation of the lungs was reported (Dyer and Esch 1976). Specific details about the HCl exposure experienced by the fire fighters were not reported in that study. Kilburn (1996) reported that residents and a police officer became acutely ill with burning and tearing eyes, burning throats, headache, chest pains, shortness of breath, and flu-like complaints following a leak of 200 gallons of hydrochloric acid from a tanker truck. Twenty-four months later, a cohort study indicated that the incidence of neurobehavioral changes and airway obstruction was higher in the exposed population than in a referent group. The lack of measurements of exposure and health effects makes interpretation of those results difficult.

Repeated Exposures

Repeated exposures to HCl gas and hydrochloric acid occur most frequently in industrial settings. The American Conference of Governmental Industrial Hygienists (ACGIH 1991) recommended a Threshold Limit Value (TLV) ceiling of 5 ppm to minimize the acute irritation associated with industrial use of HCl. The acute irritative effects of HCl are primarily limited to the concentration, rather than to the product of concentration and time, at workplace exposure levels. Experience with HCl in the workplace provides information about the potential for long-term effects occurring from exposure to low concentrations of HCl. In general, long-term pulmonary or systemic effects have not been associated with workplace exposure at low concentrations (Perry et al. 1994). Perry et al. (1994) and IARC (1992) have reviewed the results of several studies of long-term occupational exposure. In the majority of those studies, the occupational exposures were to mixed mineral-acid vapors. Prolonged occupational exposures in which HCl concentrations repeatedly exceeded 5 ppm for 5 min or more have been associated with dental erosion and tooth decay, bleeding mucous membranes in the nose and gums, and ulceration of the nasal and oral mucosa (Remijn et al. 1982). Tarlo and Broder (1989) briefly described a case of irritant-induced asthma in a 57-year-old man exposed to hydrochloric acid and phosgene for 19 years. Exposure information was not available for that case. IARC (1992) reviewed several epidemiological studies of employees in industries associated with chronic acid exposure and concluded that the evidence was inadequate for carcinogenicity in humans exposed to HCl. Neurobehavioral and chronic obstructive lung disease have not been reported in workers chronically exposed to HCl (IARC 1992).

Potentially Sensitive Populations

Children or individuals with asthma or chronic lung disease are frequently assumed to be potentially more sensitive to irritant gases than healthy adults are; however, the data supporting that position with regard to HCl exposure are limited. Boulet (1988) described a case of rapidly progressive and severe bronchospasm in a 41-year-old asthmatic male who had been cleaning a swimming pool for almost 1 hr with a product containing hydrochloric acid. The severity of his response was enough to cause hospitalization, and 1 year after the exposure, the individual continued to have marked symptoms of asthma, which were triggered by exposure to low concentrations of airborne irritants. Exposure conditions are unknown for this case. Among nine pharmaceutical employees enveloped by HCl fumes for 15 sec when a small quantity of industrial-strength HCl was accidentally released, only one of the employees, who had a prior history of chronic obstructive airways disease, developed long-term airway hyper-reactivity (Boyce and Simpson 1996). Four other employees recovered, even though they developed severe symptoms following the HCl exposure.

HCl exposures (mean ± SD) at 0.8 ± 0.09 and 1.8 ± 0.21 ppm for 45 min (including two 15-min exercise periods) did not alter the pulmonary function or ease of nasal breathing of young adults with asthma (Stevens et al. 1992). In normal healthy humans, HCl did not appear to be as irritating as other acid compounds (H_2SO_4, SO_2, or HNO_3).

Fine et al. (1987) exposed eight subjects with asthma to a pH 2 aerosol of HCl over a 3-min period. The experiment was designed to deliver relatively large and uniform isotonic particles at high concentrations through a mouthpiece. The exposure concentration was not stated; however, H_2SO_4 was tested under the same conditions, and its exposure was estimated at 10 mg/m^3. Because the predominant component of both the HCl and H_2SO_4 aerosols was water, the HCl concentration was most likely similar to that of H_2SO_4 (10 mg/m^3 or 6.7 ppm). Specific airway resistance was reduced 50% in one of the eight subjects exposed to HCl, indicating that HCl was a weak stimulus to bronchi constriction. Buffering with glycine, which was intended to cause a more persistent alteration of airway pH, resulted in a 50% increase in airway resistance in all subjects, indicating that the asthmatic subjects were more sensitive to the buffered acidity.

In a comparison of H_2SO_4 and HCl, Kamrin (1992) estimated that populations potentially sensitive to HCl might be only fivefold more sensitive than the general population.

EFFECTS IN ANIMALS

One-Time Exposure

Pulmonary Sensory Effects A decrease in respiratory rate is considered a characteristic response to upper-respiratory-tract irritation in experimental animals and has been observed in experimental animals exposed to HCl. Other indications of sensory effects have not been reported for experimental animals exposed to HCl.

Swiss-Webster mice (four per group) exposed to HCl at 40, 99, 245, 440, or 943 ppm for 10 min showed a dose-related decrease in respiratory rate at all concentrations (Barrow et al. 1977). At 99 ppm and above, the response began within the first minute of exposure and was at a plateau within 5-7 min. At 40 ppm, the decrease in respiration was seen during the second minute of exposure, the reduction in respiratory rate was minimal, and the return to baseline was rapid. At 245 ppm and above, the return to baseline was slow. The RD_{50} (concentration that decreased the respiratory rate by 50%) for HCl was calculated to be 309 ppm for a 10-min exposure.

An RD_{50} value of 560 ppm was calculated for Sprague-Dawley rats (three per group) exposed to HCl at 200-1,538 ppm for 30 min (Hartzell et al. 1985a). The HCl concentration calculated to cause a 50% decrease in respiratory minute volume was 605 ppm. The RD_{50} values indicate that the mouse (10-min RD_{50} at 309 ppm) is more sensitive than the rat (30-min RD_{50} of 560 ppm) to HCl-induced sensory irritation.

Guinea pigs also appear to be less sensitive than mice to HCl. When groups of four guinea pigs were exposed to HCl at 320, 680, 1,040, or 1,380 ppm for 30 min, it took 6 min for signs of sensory irritation (reduced respiratory rate) to appear at 320 ppm (Burleigh-Flayer et al. 1985). Sensory irritation at the higher concentrations was immediate. The mean exposure time to progress from sensory irritation to respiratory irritation was approximately an additional 13 min.

Malek and Alarie (1989) exposed guinea pigs to HCl at 107, 140, 162, and 586 ppm for up to 30 min while exercising on a running devise. Those exposed to 140 ppm or higher exhibited mild-to-severe irritation (coughing and gasping).

In contrast to mice and guinea pigs, baboons increased the respiratory rate of exposure to HCl (Kaplan 1987). Groups of three anesthetized (ketamine) juvenile baboons exposed to HCl at 5,000 or 10,000 ppm initially held their breath for 10-20 sec and then rapidly increased their respiratory rate. Animals exposed at 500 ppm also increased their respiratory rate but with a slight delay of 1-2 min, after which a plateau was quickly reached (approximately 1 min).

The order of most to least sensitive species to HCl inhalation was the mouse, guinea pig, rat, and baboon.

Effects on Respiratory Function and Morphology   Lucia et al. (1977)

exposed Swiss-Webster mice to HCl concentrations ranging from 17 to 7,279 ppm for 10 min. Twenty-four hours later, the nasal passages were examined for evidence of histological damage. Small superficial ulcers were observed in the respiratory epithelium of mice exposed at 17 ppm. At 493 ppm, the squamous epithelium of the external nares was severely damaged. At 723 ppm, more than two-thirds of the epithelium was destroyed, and at 1,973 ppm, the entire mucosa was destroyed.

Barrow et al. (1979) also exposed Swiss-Webster mice to HCl for 10 min at concentrations ranging from 20 to 20,000 ppm and found ulceration of the nasal epithelium at concentrations of 120 ppm and higher.

Stavert et al. (1991) studied the effects of HCl at 1,300 ppm (30 min) on rats breathing through their nose or through their mouth via an endotracheal tube. The nose breathers developed severe necrotizing rhinitis, and some animals had lesions in the proximal trachea. Nasal lesions were absent in the mouth-breathing rats, but inflammatory changes were present in the trachea and lungs.

Kolesar et al. (1993) exposed rats to HCl at either 1,500 or 3,000 ppm for 1 hr by nose only. Rats were sacrificed at 24 hr, 48 hr, 7 d, or 24 d after exposure and examined for organ-weight changes and for gross pathological and histopathological changes. HCl produced damage to the surface epithelium and underlying tissues at both concentrations. By day 14, the mucosa had been restored, but scar tissue was present in animals exposed at both concentrations.

In another study, groups of four to eight guinea pigs were exposed to HCl at 320, 680, 1,040, or 1,380 ppm for 30 min (Burleigh-Flayer et al. 1985). A decrease in respiratory rate and a lengthened expiratory phase were interpreted as signs of sensory irritation; an initial increase in respiratory rate followed by a decrease due to a pause following each expiration was interpreted as a sign of respiratory irritation. Two of eight animals died during exposure at 1,380 ppm. One animal in the 1,380-ppm exposure group and two of eight in the 1,040-ppm exposure group died following exposure. Following exposures, pulmonary function was evaluated at various intervals up to 15 days by exposing the animals to room air followed by challenge with 10% CO_2. The authors concluded that tidal volumes during exposure to both room air and CO_2 challenge were unaffected by HCl. However, marked decreases in respiratory rates from pre-exposure baseline rates were observed in the two highest exposure groups exposed to either room air or 10% CO_2. Those changes persisted throughout the 15-day observation period. No changes occurred in lung weights relative to body weights in any exposure group. Histopathological examination of the lungs from the group exposed to HCl at 1,040 ppm revealed inflammatory changes, including alveolitis with congestion and hemorrhage 2 days following exposure, and inflammation, hyperplasia, and mild bronchitis 15 days following exposure. No other groups were examined.

Groups of three male baboons were exposed under ketamine anesthesia to target concentrations of HCl at 500, 5,000, or 10,000 ppm for 15 min (Kaplan et al. 1988). Analytic data indicated that actual exposures were within 20% of target concentrations in all experiments except one in which the difference was approximately 30%. Respiratory rates during exposures increased from baseline rates in a dose-related fashion: approximately 30% at 500 ppm, 50% at 5,000 ppm, and 100% at 10,000 ppm. Tidal volumes were unaffected by HCl exposure. PaO_2 (arterial blood gas) decreased approximately 40% within the 15-min exposure at the two highest concentrations, but not at the lowest, and remained lower at least 10 min following the exposures before returning to baseline rates by the time of the next analysis on day 3. Pulmonary-function tests conducted 3 days and 3 months following exposures did not reveal changes relative to baseline values. The responses of animals challenged on day 3 with 10% CO_2 were no different from those challenged before HCl exposure. However, respiratory frequency seemed to increase following CO_2 challenge 3 months after HCl exposure in the 5,000- and the 10,000-ppm groups but not in the 500-ppm group.

Incapacitation and Lethality Crane et al. (1985) studied the incapacitating potential of HCl gas (2,000-100,000 ppm) in Sprague-Dawley rats while the rats were in a cylindrical cage rotating at 6 revolutions per min (rpm). The time to incapacitation was 3 hr at 2,000 ppm and 5.5 min at 94,000 ppm. Regression equations were fit to two toxicity end points (time to incapacitation and time to death) using a nonlinear least-squares technique. The model indicated that 300 ppm was a threshold for an infinitely long exposure, and 3 min was the shortest time to death at an infinite exposure concentration. Necropsy examination indicated almost total destruction of the nares and pharynx and little damage below the trachea in incapacitated rats. The response equations for incapacitation and lethality are shown below:

$$t_i = 3 + 336/(HCl - 0.3) \text{ for incapacitation;}$$
$$t_d = 3 + 411/(HCl - 0.4) \text{ for lethality.}$$

Groups of two to four guinea pigs conditioned to exercise received whole-body exposure while running in air containing HCl at 107, 140, 162, or 586 ppm (Malek and Alarie 1989). Exposures lasted for 30 min or until the guinea pigs were incapacitated (i.e., could no longer run and did not resume running). Animals exposed to HCl at 107 ppm completed the running protocol of 30 min; the other groups were incapacitated after an average of 16 min (140 ppm), 1.3 min (162 ppm), and 0.6 min (586 ppm). The low-exposure group exhibited signs of mild irritation, and the other groups showed signs of severe irritation and coughing and gasping before incapacitation. Respiratory frequency was decreased an average of 80% from sedentary baseline values in incapacitated animals. All animals in the highest exposure group died within an average of 3 min from the start of exposure. No deaths occurred in any other group, although the animals might have been observed only briefly following exposure, and any delayed effects would not have been detected. Gross pathological examinations revealed no indications of obstructed nostrils, hyperinflated lungs, or external lung hemorrhage. Histopathological examinations were not conducted. In the absence of pathological changes, the authors concluded that deaths might have resulted from enhanced protective respiratory reflexes due to exercise, resulting in increased toxicity of HCl compared with sedentary exposures.

Groups of 10 ICR-derived CF-1 mice and 10 Sprague-Dawley-derived CFE rats were exposed to either HCl gas or aerosol for 5 or 30 min to compare the toxicity of each form of the compound (Darmer et al. 1974). Analysis of the aerosols indicated that no droplets were larger than 5 μm in diameter. Animals were observed for 7 days following exposure. Gross pathological examination of animals that died during exposure revealed moderate-to-severe changes in the lungs and upper respiratory tract. Animals surviving 7 days following exposure showed pulmonary effects, including indications of alveolar damage. Unspecified histopathological changes were also observed. The LC_{50} values for exposure to HCl as an aerosol or as a gas were similar (Table D-2). For mice, the average of the two LC_{50} values at 5 min was 12,500 ppm and at 30 min was 2,400 ppm. For rats, the average of the two LC_{50} values at 5 min was 36,000 ppm and at 30 min was 5,200 ppm. Thus, the data from Darmer et al. (1974) also indicate that mice are more sensitive than rats to HCl via inhalation.

Clinical signs included brittle and discolored hair, respiratory dis-

TABLE D-2 LC_{50}s of HCl Gas and Aerosol in Rats and Mice

Animal	5-min LC_{50}, ppm		30-min LC_{50}, ppm	
	Gas	Aerosol	Gas	Aerosol
Rats	41,000	31,000	4,700	5,600
Mice	13,700	11,200	2,600	2,100

Source: Darmer et al. 1974; rounded to three significant digits. The LC_{50} values for rats and mice exposed to HCl gas for 5-min were reported by DiPasquale and Davis 1971, Higgins et al. 1972, and Darmer et al. 1974.

tress, corneal opacities, rhinorrhitis, and severe burns on exposed skin (Darmer et al. 1974). Peak mortality occurred in 24 hr, but delayed deaths were seen 3-4 days later. Exposed animals exhibited pulmonary edema of varying degrees of severity, and pulmonary hemorrhage was observed at lethal concentrations. No other details were given.

Anderson and Alarie (1980) reported an LC_{50} value (30-min exposure, 3-hr observation) of 10,137 ppm in normal mice and 1,095 ppm in trachea-cannulated mice.

Wohlslagel et al. (1976) determined LC_{50} values (1-hr exposure, 14-day observation) for CF-1 mice (1,108 ppm) and CFE rats (3,124 ppm). Concurrent exposure to alumina did not alter the LC_{50} values, and hydrogen fluoride (HF) concurrent exposure resulted only in additive effects. Necropsy of dying animals revealed pulmonary congestion and intestinal hemorrhages in rats and mice and thymic hemorrhages in rats.

Kirsch and Drabke (1982) reported a 30-min LC_{50} of about 2,500 ppm for guinea pigs. Guinea pigs affected by HCl had a high breathing rate, coughed, wheezed, had a frothy nasal discharge, frequently preened, and moved slowly.

Rabbits and guinea pigs exposed to HCl at 4,291 ppm for 30 min or 670 ppm for 6 hr died (Machle et al. 1942). Exposure of rabbits and guinea pigs at 3,687 ppm for 5 min was the highest concentration that produced no deaths. The longest exposure of rabbits and guinea pigs that resulted in no deaths was 6 hr per day for 5 days at 67 ppm.

Hartzell et al. (1985b) determined the 5-, 10-, 15-, 22.5-, 30-, and 60-min LC_{50} values for HCl gas in male Sprague-Dawley rats to be 15,900, 8,370, 6,920, 5,920, 3,715, and 2,810 ppm, respectively. $L(CT)_{50}$ (the product of concentration and time that results in death of 50% of the test animals) values for HCl (Table D-3) vary from approximately 80,000 ppm·min (5-min exposure at approximately 16,000 ppm) at approxi-

TABLE D-3 L(CT)$_{50}$ Values for Rats Exposed to HCl Gas

Exposure Duration, min	L(CT)$_{50}$ Value, ppm·min	95% Confidence Interval, ppm·min
5	79,500	57,700-109,400
10	83,700	77,700-90,100
15	103,800	50,700-133,500
22.5	133,200	77,800-228,300
30	111,450	76,200-163,000
60	168,600	135,000-210,700

Source: Hartzell et al. 1985b.

mately 170,000 ppm·min (60-min exposure at approximately 2,800 ppm).

MacEwen and Vernot (1974) combined the data from Darmer et al. (1974) with their own 60-min-LC$_{50}$ HCl-vapor data and calculated L(CT)$_{50}$ values for rats and mice (Table D-4). They concluded that Haber's law appeared to be applicable to HCl for those exposure times.

Ocular Effects Mice exposed to HCl vapor for 10 min were studied for ocular effects (GEOMET Technologies 1981). Significant inflammatory cell infiltrations were observed at 490 ppm in the palpebral and ocular conjunctivae. Corneal necrosis and inflammatory cell infiltrates in the eyelids were observed at 1,074 ppm. Extensive damage to the eye and eyelids was seen at a concentration of 1,946 ppm and above.

Swiss-Webster mice were exposed to HCl at 20-20,000 ppm for 10 min (Barrow et al. 1979). Ocular damage indicated by polymorphonuclear leukocyte infiltration of the conjunctiva was observed in animals exposed to HCl at 480 ppm, corneal necrosis was observed at 700 ppm, and severe damage to the globes was observed at 3,000 ppm.

TABLE D-4 Comparison of L(CT)$_{50}$ Values for Rats and Mice Exposed to HCl Gas

Animals	L(CT)$_{50}$, ppm·min		
	5-min	30-min	60-min
Rats	204,945	141,030	187,440
Mice	68,725	79,320	66,480

Source: MacEwen and Vernot 1974.

Corneal opacities were observed in all five guinea pigs exposed to HCl at 1,380 ppm, in four of six guinea pigs exposed at 1,040 ppm, and in one of four guinea pigs exposed at 680 ppm (Burleigh-Flayer et al. 1985). Corneal opacity was not observed in guinea pigs exposed at 320 ppm.

Ocular damage appears to occur at similar HCl concentrations in mice and guinea pigs. The no-effect level for ocular damage appears to be at 400-500 ppm.

Neurobehavioral Effects   Single baboons were exposed to HCl at 190, 810, 890, 2,780, 11,400, 16,570, or 17,290 ppm for 5 min (Kaplan 1987). The animals had been conditioned to a relatively simple escape-performance test designed to simulate human escape performance, which was begun after the 5-min exposure. An increase occurred in the number of attempts to escape after exposure compared with that before exposure, indicating an irritative response in the animals. Escape attempts increased at 190 ppm. Other signs of irritation were coughing and frothing at the mouth at 810 ppm, progressing to profuse salivation, blinking and rubbing the eyes, and head-shaking at higher concentrations. The animals exposed at 16,570 and 17,290 ppm exhibited severe dyspnea that persisted after exposure, followed by death several weeks later from bacterial infections. Histopathological examination of those animals revealed pneumonia, pulmonary edema, and tracheitis with epithelial erosion.

Kaplan et al. (1984) used an operant test (shuttle box) to evaluate escape performance in rats exposed to HCl. Rats were exposed for 5 min at concentrations ranging from 11,800 to 87,660 ppm. At concentrations up to 76,730 ppm, but not at 87,660 ppm, the rats were able to escape. Rats exposed at 11,800 and 14,410 did not die, but those exposed at 15,250 ppm and higher died after exposure and the rat exposed at the highest concentration died during exposure.

Developmental and Reproductive Toxicities

Rats received a single 1-hr exposure to HCl at 300 ppm either 12 days before mating or on day 9 of pregnancy (Pavlova 1976). Signs of severe dyspnea and cyanosis were noted and one-third of the rats died. Embryo and fetal toxicity was observed; the toxicity appeared to be secondary to severe maternal pulmonary effects.

One-Time Exposures—Combined Exposures Simulating Sensitive Populations

Higgins et al. (1972) exposed mice and rats to carbon monoxide (CO) at concentrations sufficient to produce 25% carboxyhemoglobin (1,500 ppm for mice and 2,100 ppm for rats) and determined 7-day LC_{50} values for HCl. The LC_{50} values for HCl without exposure to CO (13,700 ppm for mice and 41,000 ppm for rats) were not significantly different from the combined HCl-CO exposure (10,700 ppm for mice and 39,000 ppm for rats). Dipasquale and Davis (1971) showed that a CO exposure sufficient to induce 25% carboxyhemoglobin (CO at 2,100 ppm in rats and 1,500 ppm in mice) had no effect on 5-min LC_{50} values in Wistar rats and ICR mice.

Hartzell et al. (1985a) developed a mathematical model describing the intoxication of rats with CO. They found that HCl exposure modified the CO-induced intoxication of rats only slightly and only within a "window" of exposure concentrations of HCl at about 400 to 1,000 ppm and CO at less than 4,000 ppm.

Tables D-5 and D-6 provide additional information on acute toxicity studies conducted with HCl.

Repeated Exposures

A group of Swiss-Webster mice was exposed to HCl at 309 ppm (the RD_{50}) for 6 hr per day (Buckley et al. 1984). After three exposures, all the mice were dead or were moribund, and exposures were discontinued. Histopathological examination revealed severe exfoliation, erosion, ulceration, and necrosis of the nasal respiratory epithelium but only slight-to-mild changes in the squamous epithelium and olfactory epithelium. No changes were observed in the lower respiratory tract.

The NRC (1987) reviewed the data on repeated exposures of experimental animals to HCl and concluded that the primary effect was upper respiratory irritation. Rats and mice were exposed to HCl at 10, 20, or 50 ppm for 6 hr per day, 5 days per week for 90 days (Toxigenics 1984). Histopathological examination revealed minimal-to-mild rhinitis in exposed rats, and cheilitis and very mild degenerative changes in the nasal turbinates of all exposed mice. The degenerative changes were typical of those seen following exposure to many irritants and are considered reversible following cessation of exposure.

TABLE D-5 Toxicity Studies of HCl in Experimental Animals

Species	Exposure Duration	Exposure Concentration, ppm	Effect Concentration, ppm[1]	End Points and Comments	References
Pulmonary sensory effects					
One-Time Exposures					
Mouse, Swiss-Webster	10 min	40, 99, 245, 440, 943	40 309	- Decreased respiratory rate at 2 min of exposure—effect minimal and rapidly reversible - Calculated RD_{50} (219-435 ppm 95% CI)	Barrow et al. 1977
Mouse, Swiss-Webster	10 min	20-20,000	50	Decreased respiratory rate	Barrow et al. 1979
Rat, Sprague-Dawley	30 min	200, 295, 784, 1,006, 1,538	560	30-min RD_{50}; exposure-related decrease in respiratory frequency and minute volume; maximum effect within 2 min of start of exposure; 605 ppm caused a 50% decrease in respiratory minute volume	Hartzell et al. 1985a
Guinea pig, 4-8/group	30 min, no exercise	320, 680, 1,040, 1,380	320 680	- Decreased respiratory rate after 6 min of exposure - Immediate decrease in respiratory rate	Burleigh-Flayer et al. 1985
Guinea pig, 2-4/group	30 min, with exercise	107, 140, 162, 586	140	Mild-to-severe irritation, cough, gasping	Malek and Alarie 1989
Baboon, 3/group	15 min, anesthetized	500, 5,000, 10,000	500 5,000	- Increased respiratory rate after 1-2 min - Held breath for 10-20 sec, then rapidly increased respiratory rate	Kaplan 1987

Respiratory Function and Morphology

Species	Duration	Concentration	Effects	Reference
Mouse, Swiss-Webster	10 min	17–7,279	17 493	- Superficial ulcers of respiratory epithelium - Severe damage to squamous epithelium of external nares	Lucia et al. 1977
			723 1,973	- More than two-thirds of epithelium destroyed - Entire mucosa destroyed	
Mouse, Swiss-Webster	10 min	20–20,000	>50 120 7,000	- Decreased respiratory rate - Ulceration of nasal epithelium - Complete destruction of nasal bone	Barrow et al. 1979
Rat	30 min	1,300	1,300	Breathed HCl through nose or endotracheal tube; nasal breathers had rhinitis and proximal tracheitis; tube breathers had tracheitis and pneumonitis (histopathological examination 24 hr later)	Stavert et al. 1991
Rat	1 hr	1,500, 3,000	1,500	Damage to surface epithelium of the nasal mucosa; mucosa restored by 14 d but scar tissue present (histopathological examination at 24 hr, 48 hr, 7 d, and 14 d)	Kolesar et al. 1993
Guinea pig, 4–8/group	30 min	320, 680, 1,040, 1,380	1,040	Marked decrease in respiratory rate (2/8 died); lung histopathology revealed inflammatory changes 2 and 15 d post-exposure; marked decrease in respiratory rates on challenge with CO_2 exposure, but tidal volumes not affected	Burleigh-Flayer et al. 1985
Baboon, 3/group	15 min, anesthetized	500, 5,000, 10,000	500 5,000 10,000	- 30% increase in respiratory rate - 50% increase in respiratory rate - 100% increase in respiratory rate	Kaplan et al. 1988

TABLE D-5 Toxicity Studies of HCl in Experimental Animals *(Continued)*

Species	Exposure Duration	Exposure Concentration, ppm	Effect Concentration, ppm[1]	End Points and Comments	References
Baboon, 3/group	15 min, anesthetized	500, 5,000, 10,000	≥5,000	PaO_2 decreased 40% and possible long-term effects; respiratory frequency seemed to increase following CO_2 challenge 3 mo after exposure	Kaplan et al. 1988
Incapacitation					
Rat, Sprague-Dawley	Until incapacitation	2,000-100,000	2,000 94,000	- 3 hr until incapacitation - 5.5 min until incapacitation (see also Table D-6)	Crane et al. 1985
Guinea pig	Until incapacitation	107-586	107 140 162 586	- All ran full 30 min - Average 16 min until incapacitation - Average 1.3 min - Average 0.6 min (all died within an average of 3 min) (see also Table D-6)	Malek and Alarie 1989
Lethality					
Mouse, CF-1, 10/group (gas)	5 min 30 min	(see Table D-6)	≈13,700 ≈2,600	- 5-min LC_{50} (≈10,300-18,300 ppm, 95% CI) - 30-min LC_{50} (≈2,300-3,100 ppm, 95% CI)	Darmer et al. 1974
Mouse, CF-1, 10/group (aerosol)	5 min 30 min	(see Table D-6)	≈11,200 ≈2,100	- 5-min LC_{50} (≈10,000-12,500 ppm, 95% CI) - 30-min LC_{50} (≈1,800-2,600 ppm, 95% CI)	Darmer et al. 1974
Rat, CFE, 10/group (gas)	5 min 30 min	(see Table D-6)	≈41,000 ≈4,700	- 5-min LC_{50} (≈34,800-48,300 ppm, 95% CI) - 30-min LC_{50} (≈4,100-5,400 ppm, 95% CI)	Darmer et al. 1974
Rat, CFE, 10/group (aerosol)	5 min 30 min	(see Table D-6)	≈31,000 ≈5,700	- 5-min LC_{50} (≈26,800-35,800 ppm, 95% CI) - 30-min LC_{50} (≈4,600-6,600 ppm, 95% CI)	Darmer et al. 1974

Species	Duration	Concentration	Notes	Reference
Mouse	30 min	10,137	30-min LC_{50}; 3-hr post exposure	Anderson and Alarie 1980
Mouse	30 min	1,095	30-min LC_{50}; 3-hr post exposure; tracheal-cannulated mice	Anderson and Alarie 1980
Mouse, female CF-1 (ICR derived)	60 min	(see Table D-6)	≈1,100	60-min LC_{50}; 14-d post-exposure (≈870–1,400 ppm, 95% CI)	Wohlslagel et al. 1976
Rat, male CFE (Sprague-Dawley derived)	60 min	(see Table D-6)	≈3,100	60-min LC_{50}; 14-d observation (≈2,800–3,500 ppm, 95% CI)	Wohlslagel et al. 1976
Guinea pig 8/group	30 min	(see Table D-6)	≈2,500	30-min LC_{50}	Kirsch and Drabke 1982
Rat, Sprague-Dawley, male	5 min 10 min 15 min 22.5 min 30 min 60 min	15,900 8,370 6,920 5,920 3,715 2,810	-5-min LC_{50} -10-min LC_{50} -15-min LC_{50} -22.5-min LC_{50} -30-min LC_{50} -60-min LC_{50}	Hartzell et al. 1985b
Guinea pig, 4-8/group	30 min, no exercise	320, 680, 1,040, 1,380	- 2/8 died after exposure - 2/8 died during exposure, 1/8 after exposure	Burleigh-Flayer et al. 1985
Baboon, 1 at each level	5 min	190, 810, 890, 2,780, 11,400, 16,750, 17,290	16,750	Delayed deaths	Kaplan 1987

123

TABLE D-5 Toxicity Studies of HCl in Experimental Animals *(Continued)*

Species	Exposure Duration	Exposure Concentration, ppm	Effect Concentration, ppm[1]	End Points and Comments	References
Ocular Toxicity					
Mouse (vapor)	10 min	490-3,062	490 1,074 1,946 3,062	- Conjunctival PMN leukocyte infiltrates - Corneal necrosis; infiltrates in lids - Extensive ocular damage - Rupture of the globe	GEOMET Technologies 1981
Mouse, Swiss-Webster	10 min	20-20,000	480 700 3,000	- Conjunctival PMN leukocyte infiltrates - Corneal necrosis - Severe damage to the globes	Barrow et al. 1979
Guinea pig, male	30 min	320, 680, 1,040, 1380	680	Corneal opacity; see Table D-6 for summary of exposure-response	Burleigh-Flayer et al. 1985
Neurobehavioral Effects					
Baboon, 1/group	5 min	190, 810, 890, 2,780, 11,400, 16,570, 17,290	190 810 890 16,570	- Increased number of escape attempts - Coughing and frothing at the mouth - Profuse salivation, blinking, head-shaking - Severe dyspnea, followed by death from bacterial infection	Kaplan 1987
Rat	5 min	11,800-87,660	87,660	Unable to escape (all rats exposed at lower concentrations performed escape task; however, all rats exposed at more than 14,410 ppm died)	Kaplan et al. 1984

Combined Exposures Simulating Sensitive Populations

Species	Duration	Concentration (ppm)	Effects	Reference
Mouse, ICR	5 min	(see Table D-6)	≈13,800 5-min LC_{50}; 7-d post-exposure	Higgins et al. 1972; DiPasquale and Davis 1971
Mouse, ICR	5 min	Unspecified range	≈10,700 5-min LC_{50}; 7-d post-exposure; combined with CO at 1,500 ppm	Higgins et al. 1972
Rat, Wistar	5 min	(see Table D-6)	≈41,000 5-min LC_{50}; 7-d post-exposure.	Higgins et al. 1972; DiPasquale and Davis 1971
Rat, Wistar	5 min	Unspecified range	≈39,000 5-min LC_{50}; 7-d post-exposure; combined with CO at 2,100 ppm	Higgins et al. 1972

Repeated Exposures

Species	Duration	Concentration (ppm)	Effects	Reference
Mouse	6 hr/d, 1-3 d	309	All mice died or were moribund by third exposure; severe irritation of nasal respiratory epithelium; slight-to-moderate changes in olfactory epithelium; no changes in lower respiratory tract.	Buckley et al. 1984
Guinea pig, rabbit, monkey	6 hr/d, 5 d/wk, 28 d	34	No immediate effects and no gross pathological lesions	Machle et al. 1942
Guinea pig	2 hr/d, 28 d	0.1	No lung irritation	Kirsch and Drabke 1982
Rat	6 hr/d, 5 d/wk, 90 d	0, 10, 20, 50	Dose-related rhinitis ranging from minimal to mild beginning at 10 ppm	Toxigenics 1984

TABLE D-5 Toxicity Studies of HCl in Experimental Animals *(Continued)*

Species	Exposure Duration	Exposure Concentration, ppm	Effect Concentration, ppm[a]	End Points and Comments	References
Mouse	6 hr/d, 5 d/wk, 90 d	0, 10, 20, 50	10	Eosinophilic globules in epithelial cells of the nasal turbinates; reversible sign of very mild degeneration	Toxigenics 1984
Rat	6 hr/d, 5 d/wk, lifetime	10	10	Increased incidence of laryngeal and tracheal hyperplasia, but no evidence of HCl-induced tumors	Sellakumar et al. 1985; Albert et al. 1982

[a] Number of significant digits listed are as reported in original reports, unless the value is preceded by ≈, which indicates that the value has been rounded to the nearest 100th ppm.

Abbreviations: RD_{50}, concentration that produces a 50% decrease in respiratory rate; CI, confidence interval; LC_{50}, concentration lethal to 50% of the test animals; PMN, polymorphonuclear.

TABLE D-6 Summary of Exposure-Response Data for HCl Gas (Except as Noted)

Species	Exposure Duration	Exposure Concentration, ppm	Effect Level	End Points and Comments	References
Guinea pig, male (English Smooth Hair)	30 min	0 320 680 1,040 1,380	0/4 0/4 1/4 4/6 5/5	Corneal opacity	Burleigh-Flayer et al. 1985
Guinea pig, male (English Smooth Hair)	30 min	0 320 680 1,040 1,380	0/4 0/4 0/4 2/8 3/8	Mortality	Burleigh-Flayer et al. 1985
Baboon, male	15 min	500 5,000 10,000	See refs. for graphs of results	Respiratory and blood-gas measurements; baboon and rat lethality data available in Kaplan et al. 1984; also see Kaplan et al. 1987 for lack of effect of HCl in avoidance and escape behavior	Kaplan et al. 1988

TABLE D-6 Summary of Exposure-Response Data for HCl Gas (Except as Noted) *(Continued)*

Species	Exposure Duration	Exposure Concentration, ppm	Effect Level	End Points and Comments	References
Mouse, CF-1 (ICR derived)	5 min	3,200	1/10	Mortality; 5-min LC_{50} = 13,745 ppm (10,333-18,283, 95% CI); clinical signs not assigned to concentrations	Darmer et al. 1974
		5,060	1/10		
		6,145	2/10		
		6,410	0/10		
		7,525	6/10		
		8,065	2/10		
		9,276	5/10		
		13,655	6/10		
		26,485	13/15		
		30,000	13/15		
Mouse, CF-1 (ICR derived)	30 min	410	0/15	Mortality; 30-min LC_{50} = 2,644 ppm (2,264-3,086 ppm, 95% CI); clinical signs not assigned to concentrations	Darmer et al. 1974
		1,134	2/15		
		2,678	8/15		
		2,721	4/15		
		2,942	12/15		
		3,071	6/15		
		4,045	11/15		
		4,076	13/15		
		5,363	14/15		

Species	Duration	Concentration (ppm)	Mortality	Effects	Reference
Mouse, CF-1 (ICR derived)	5 min	9,058 10,059 12,104 14,913 17,000 18,773	3/10 3/10 5/10 9/10 9/10 10/10	Mortality; 5-min LC_{50} = 11,238 ppm (10,006–12,547 ppm, 95% CI)	Darmer et al. 1974 Note: HCl Aerosol
Mouse CF-1 (ICR derived)	30 min	1,204 2,127 2,557 2,720 2,910 3,036 4,432	2/10 5/10 5/10 5/10 9/10 7/10 10/10	Mortality; 30-min LC_{50} = 2,142 ppm (1,779–2,580 ppm, 95% CI)	Darmer et al. 1974 Note: HCl Aerosol
Rat, CFE (Sprague-Dawley derived)	5 min	30,000 32,255 39,850 45,200 57,290	0/10 1/10 6/10 7/10 9/10	Mortality; 5-min LC_{50} = 40,989 ppm (34,803–48,272 ppm, 95% CI)	Darmer et al. 1974
Rat, CFE (Sprague-Dawley derived)	30 min	2,078 2,678 3,071 5,180 6,068 6,681	0/10 1/10 0/10 5/10 8/10 10/10	Mortality; 30-min LC_{50} = 4,701 ppm (4,129–5,352 ppm, 95% CI)	Darmer et al. 1974

TABLE D-6 Summary of Exposure-Response Data for HCl Gas (Except as Noted) (Continued)

Species	Exposure Duration	Exposure Concentration, ppm	Effect Level	End Points and Comments	References
Rat, CFE (Sprague-Dawley derived)	5 min	6,571 19,312 25,324 29,648 38,746 40,810 62,042	0/10 1/10 3/10 6/10 6/10 7/10 10/10	Mortality; 5-min LC_{50} = 31,008 ppm (26,824-35,845 ppm, 95% CI); clinical signs not assigned to concentrations	Darmer et al. 1974 Note: HCl Aerosol
Rat, CFE (Sprague-Dawley derived)	30 min	2,910 4,481 6,078 6,640	1/10 0/10 6/8 8/10	Mortality; 30-min LC_{50} = 5,666 ppm (4,555-6,614 ppm, 95% CI); clinical signs not assigned to concentrations	Darmer et al. 1974 Note: HCl Aerosol
Rat, Sprague-Dawley (n = 42-43)	5.5 min to 3 hr	2,000-100,000	See equations	Response equations for incapacitation, T_i = 3 + 336/(HCl - 0.3); for lethality, T_d = 3 + 441/HCl - 0.4)	Crane et al. 1985
Guinea pig, outbred English short hair				Time to incapacitation (min) Distance traveled (m) Deaths	Malek and Alarie 1989
		107	0/3	>30 795 0/3	
		140	3/3	16.5 ± 8.6 437 ± 229 0/3	
		162	3/3	1.3 ± 0.9 47.8 ± 7.4 0/3	
		586	3/3	0.65 ± 0.08 17.1 ± 2.2 3/3	

Rat, Sprague-Dawley, male	5 min	9,200 10,785 12,584 14,307 15,459 20,300	0/6 3/6 2/6 0/6 3/6 6/6	Mortality; 5-min LC_{50} = 15,900 ppm (11,540-21,890 ppm, 95% CI); 14-d observation	Hartzell et al. 1985b
Rat, Sprague-Dawley, male	10 min	5,444 7,629 8,114 8,425 9,170	0/6 1/6 5/8 1/8 6/6	Mortality; 10-min LC_{50} = 8,370 ppm (7,770-9,010 ppm, 95% CI); 14-d observation	Hartzell et al. 1985b
Rat, Sprague-Dawley, male	15 min	4,360 6,171 7,980 8,960 9,990	0/6 3/6 4/6 4/6 6/6	Mortality; 15-min LC_{50} = 6,920 ppm (5,380-8,900 ppm, 95% CI); 14-d observation	Hartzell et al. 1985b
Rat, Sprague-Dawley, male	22.5 min	4,864 6,414 7,487 8,103 8,646 10,137	2/6 4/6 6/6 2/6 4/6 6/6	Mortality; 22.5-min LC_{50} = 5,920 ppm (3,455-10,145 ppm, 95% CI); 14-d observation	Hartzell et al. 1985b
Rat, Sprague-Dawley, male	30 min	2,610 3,713 4,090 5,776 6,470 8,280	2/6 4/6 1/6 8/8 4/6 6/6	Mortality; 30-min LC_{50} = 3,715 ppm (2,540-5,435 ppm, 95% CI);	Hartzell et al. 1985b

TABLE D-6 Summary of Exposure-Response Data for HCl Gas (Except as Noted) (*Continued*)

Species	Exposure Duration	Exposure Concentration, ppm	Effect Level	End Points and Comments	References
Rat, Sprague-Dawley, male	60 min	1,793 2,281 2,600 4,277 4,460 4,854	0/6 3/6 1/6 7/8 6/6 6/6	Mortality; 60-min LC_{50} = 2,810 ppm (2,250-3,510 ppm, 95% CI)	Hartzell et al. 1985b
Mouse, CF-1 (ICR derived), female	60 min	557 985 1,387 1,902 2,476	2/10 3/10 6/10 8/10 10/10	Mortality; 60-min LC_{50} = 1,108 ppm (874-1,404 ppm, 95% CI)	Wohlslagel et al. 1976
Rat, CFE (Sprague-Dawley derived), male	60 min	1,813 2,585 3,274 3,941 4,455	0/10 2/10 6/10 8/10 10/10	Mortality; 60-min LC_{50} = 3,124 ppm (2,829-3,450 ppm, 95% CI)	Wohlslagel et al. 1976
Guinea pig	30 min	1,309 1,538 2,125 4,082 5,708	0/8 1/8 3/8 7/8 8/8	Mortality; 30-min LC_{50} = 2,519 ppm	Kirsch and Drabke 1982

Species	Duration	Concentration (ppm)	Mortality	Effects	Reference
Mouse, IRC, 15/group	5 min	3,200	1/15	Mortality; 5-min LC_{50} = 13,745 ppm (10,333-18,283 ppm, 95% CI); 7-d observation	Higgins et al. 1972
		5,060	1/15		
		6,145	2/15		
		6,410	0/15		
		7,525	6/15		
		8,065	2/15		
		9,276	5/15		
		13,655	6/15		
		26,485	13/15		
		30,000	13/15		
Rat, Wistar 10/group	5 min	30,000	0/10	Mortality; 5-min LC_{50} = 40,989 ppm (34,803-48,272 ppm, 95% CI); 7-d observation	Higgins et al. 1972
		32,000	1/10		
		39,850	6/10		
		45,200	7/10		
		57,290	9/10		

Abbreviations: CI, confidence interval; LC_{50}, concentration lethal to 50% of the test animals.

Rabbits (three per group), guinea pigs (three per group), and a monkey exposed to HCl at 34 ppm for 6 hr per day, 5 days per week for 4 weeks showed no immediate effects and no gross pathological lesions (Machle et al. 1942).

Guinea pigs exposed to HCl at 0.1 ppm for 2 hr per day for 4 weeks showed no effects on lung irritation (Kirsch and Drabke 1982).

Rats receiving a lifetime exposure at 10 ppm for 6 hr per day, 5 days per week developed a higher incidence of laryngeal and tracheal hyperplasia than controls but showed no evidence of HCl-induced tumors (Sellakumar et al. 1985; Albert et al. 1982).

IARC (1992) reviewed the study reported by Sellakumar et al. (1985) and single-exposure studies showing that HCl induced chromosomal aberrations and mutations in mammalian cells in vitro and concluded that the evidence was inadequate to conclude that HCl was carcinogenic in experimental animals.

ESTABLISHED INHALATION EXPOSURE LIMITS

Figure D-1 and Table D-7 list inhalation exposure limits established by various groups. ACGIH established a Threshold Limit Value (TLV) ceiling of 5 ppm in 1963. The TLV was recommended to minimize potential toxicity and acute irritation associated with occupational exposure to HCl (ACGIH 1991). Between 1946 and 1947, the ACGIH TLV for HCl was 10 ppm as a time-weighted average (TWA); in 1948, it was lowered to 5 ppm as a TWA. In 1963, ACGIH changed the 5-ppm recommendation from a TWA to a ceiling value because of reports of respiratory irritation from short-term exposures to HCl at 5 ppm and above (permissible as long as the average concentration over the 8-hr work day did not exceed 5 ppm). The Occupational Safety and Health Administration (OSHA) also established a permissible exposure limit (PEL) as a ceiling value of 5 ppm. The occupational exposure limits (OELs) recommended by ACGIH, OSHA, various other state and federal agencies, and agencies in other countries have been based more on human experience than on animal test data.

Table D-8 shows inhalation exposure guidelines for HCl recommended by previous NRC committees. The NRC (1987) derived a 10-min EEGL for HCl of 100 ppm by applying uncertainty factors of 10 for species differences and 0.64 for paucity of data to the 10-min RD_{50} in

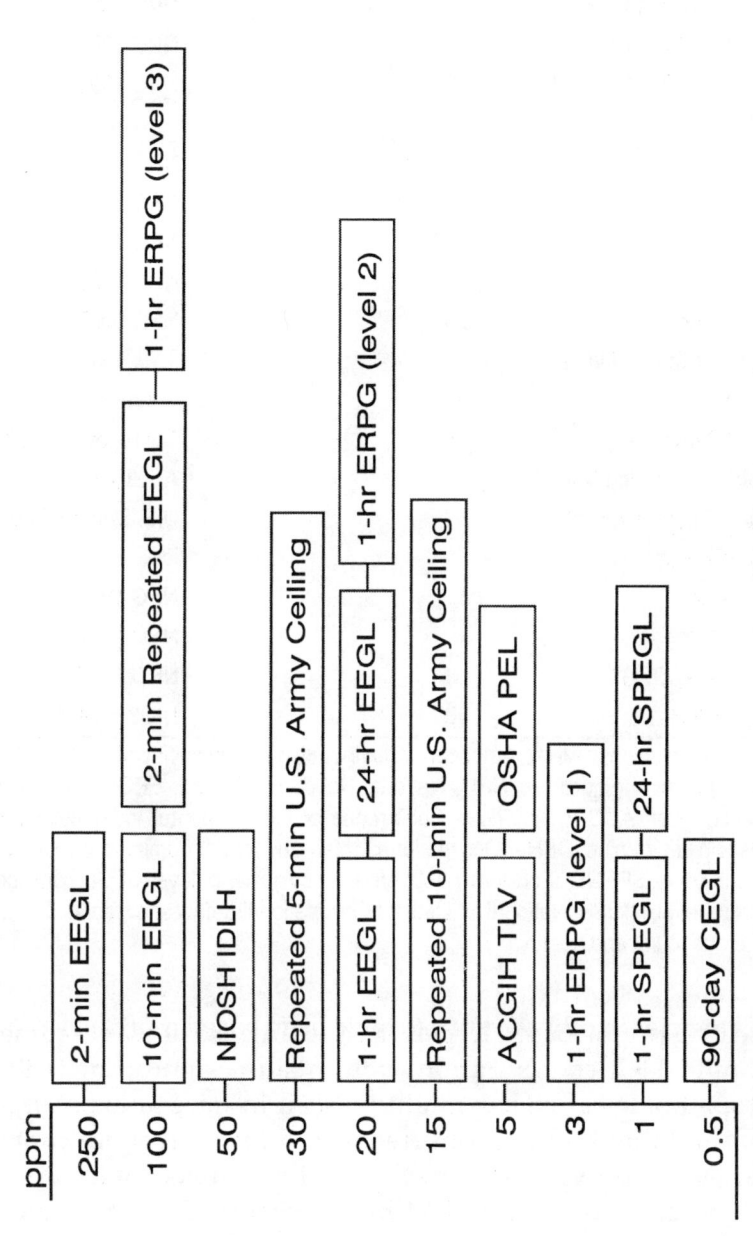

FIGURE D-1 Currently recommended exposure limits for HCl (see Table D-7 for abbreviations and sources).

TABLE D-7 Currently Recommended Exposure Limits for HCl

Exposure Limit	Concentration, ppm	Reference
AIHA ERPGs		
Level 1, 1 hr	3	NRC 1991
Level 2, 1 hr	20	NRC 1991
Level 3, 1 hr	100	NRC 1991
NRC EEGLs		
2 min	250	NRC 1991
2 min repeated	100	NRC 1991
10 min	100	NRC 1987
1 hr	20	NRC 1987
24 hr	20	NRC 1987
U.S. Army Ceiling Limits		
5 min	30	Cohen et al. 1982
60 min	15	Cohen et al. 1982
ACGIH TLV, ceiling limit	5	ACGIH 1991
OSHA PEL, ceiling limit	5	U.S. Dept. of Labor 1998
NRC SPEGLs		
1 hr	1	NRC 1987
24 hr	1	NRC 1987
NRC 90-day CEGL	0.5	NRC 1987
NIOSH IDLH	50	NIOSH 1994

Abbreviations: AIHA, American Industrial Hygiene Association; ERPG, emergency response planning guidelines; NRC, National Research Council; EEGL, emergency exposure guidance level; ACGIH, American Conference of Governmental Industrial Hygienists; TLV, Threshold Limit Value; OSHA, Occupational Safety and Health Administration; PEL, permissible exposure level; SPEGL, short-term public emergency guidance level; CEGL, continuous exposure guidance level; NIOSH, National Institute for Occupational Safety and Health; IDLH, immediately dangerous to life and health.

mice (309 ppm). Based largely on data in mice, it was assumed that the 100-ppm HCl concentration would cause significant irritation, that histopathological effects might be seen in mice at exposures near the RD_{50}, and that higher exposures would result in significant persistent injuries to the respiratory tract. The NRC applied an uncertainty factor of 20 to both the 1-hr and 24-hr emergency exposure guidance level

TABLE D-8 Previously Recommended Inhalation Exposure Guidelines by the National Research Council

HCl Concentration, ppm

Exposure Duration	1965	1971	1971	1972	1977	1987	1991
2 min							250 (EEGL)
10 min	30 (EEL)	7 (PEL)	4 (STPL)		100 (EEL)	100 (EEGL)	100 (EEGL)
30 min	20 (EEL)	3 (PEL)	2 (STPL)		50 (EEL)		
1 hr	10 (EEL)	3 (PEL)	2 (STPL)	5 (EEL)	20 (EEGL)	20 (EEGL) 1 (SPEGL)	
24 hr						20 (EEGL) 1 (SPEGL)	
90 d				1 (CEL)		0.5 (CEGL)	

Source: Modified from NRC 1987 and 1991.
Abbreviations: EEGL, emergency exposure guidance level; EEL, emergency exposure limit; PEL, permissible exposure level; STPL, short-term public limit; SPEGL, short-term public emergency guidance level; CEL, continuous exposure limit; CEGL, continuous exposure guidance level.

(EEGL) values to derive the 1-hr and 24-hr short-term public emergency guidance level (SPEGL) values of 1 ppm to protect sensitive populations. A 90-day continuous emergency guidance level (CEGL) was derived from subchronic inhalation studies with rats and mice that showed that 50 ppm produced minimal effects (NRC 1987). An uncertainty factor of 100 was applied to the 50-ppm exposure concentration to derive the 0.5-ppm 90-day CEGL.

In 1991, the NRC recommended 2-min EEGLs for single (500 ppm) and multiple (100 ppm) exposures to HCl. These recommendations were based primarily on data showing that baboons exposed to HCl at 500 ppm for 15 min exhibited signs of irritation but did not show changes in hypoxia or pulmonary function and were able to perform escape tasks. The multiple-exposure EEGL for HCl was derived from those data by applying an uncertainty factor of 5.

EVALUATION OF TOXICITY INFORMATION

HCl is a potentially severe respiratory-tract irritant in humans. However, the irritating properties of HCl prevent more than transient voluntary exposure to concentrations that are likely to cause serious adverse effects.

As indicated in the previous section, data from rodent models have been used to establish short-term exposure guidelines for HCl and to gain a perspective on the mechanisms and effects of high-concentration short-term exposures. Following exposure to high concentrations of HCl, rodents exhibit signs of sensory and respiratory irritation. Sensory irritation is evoked by stimulation of trigeminal nerve endings in the nasal passages, whereas respiratory irritation occurs through contact of HCl with the lower respiratory tract. As HCl is inhaled, the highly soluble gas (or aerosol) readily dissolves in the mucosal lining of the nasal passages. When the "scrubbing" mechanism of the mucosal lining is overwhelmed at high concentrations, HCl enters the lower respiratory tract. Thus, at a given concentration, a delay occurs between the onset of signs of sensory irritation and signs of respiratory irritation. In rodents, each type of irritation shows a specific threshold and dose-response curve. Each type of irritation can be detected by monitoring respiratory patterns.

In some guinea pig studies, lethality occurred following moderately high HCl exposures without obvious gross pathological causes. Protective respiratory mechanisms exacerbated by exercise in the guinea pigs might have been the proximate cause of lethality among the animals acutely exposed to moderately high HCl concentrations. That view is supported by observations that even though significant pathological effects occurred in the nasal passages of rodents following HCl exposures, no effects occurred in the lower respiratory tract except at high concentrations.

Mice appear to be much more sensitive to the lethal effects of HCl than rats, guinea pigs, rabbits, or baboons. To some extent, this increased sensitivity might be due to a less effective scrubbing mechanism that would remove HCl in the upper respiratory tract. The data suggest that mice might not be an appropriate model for extrapolation to humans; however, rodent studies often provide the only data sets large enough for statistical model development.

Recent studies have demonstrated significant differences between primates and rodents in their responses to HCl exposure. Exposure of rodents to HCl produces dose-related decreases in respiratory frequency and increases in pauses between breaths, changes that are interpreted as protective mechanisms. Baboons exposed at concentrations of up to 17,000 ppm for 5 min, however, exhibited increases in respiratory frequency that could be interpreted as a compensatory mechanism in response to hypoxia. Moreover, conditioned baboons were able to perform tasks at those high concentrations. Although concentrations above 11,000 ppm produced delayed death, concentrations up to 500 ppm did not produce permanent respiratory-function impairment.

Although some human subpopulations are presumed to have a greater sensitivity to respiratory irritants such as HCl (Chapter 3), no data are available for HCl that directly support this hypothesis. Data for adults with mild asthma do not indicate that this population has an unusual sensitivity to HCl; however, data for moderate-to-high exposure concentrations and for more severely affected individuals are not available. Animal models using concurrent exposure to CO to induce levels of 25% carboxyhemoglobin in the blood do not support the hypothesis that hypoxia is an additional risk factor of concern for HCl exposure.

There are mechanistic considerations that suggest that asthmatic individuals could be more sensitive to acidic respiratory irritants (Spengler et al. 1990). Although the pH of tracheobronchial mucus is nearly neutral in healthy people, mucus pH is more acidic in those with asthma. As mucus becomes more acidic, its viscosity increases, resulting in increased airway resistance and decreased mucociliary clearance. Ciliary motion stops and epithelial cells die as mucus pH approaches 4.9. Because the mucociliary apparatus in asthmatic individuals is typically impaired or severely degraded, small changes in mucus pH might have significant consequences. Some of these responses have been observed in experimental animals exposed to H_2SO_4, but so far, similar effects due to HCl have not been reported.

The studies by Stevens et al. (1992) and Fine et al. (1987) suggest that the sensitivity of asthmatic individuals to HCl might not be as great as previously thought. The reasons for that are not clear, but an important protective mechanism might be the buffering capacity of the oral and nasopharyngeal regions. If HCl is adequately buffered in the upper airways, substantial exposure of the more sensitive lower airways of asthmatic individuals might not occur. Thus, although it might be prudent to apply a "safety factor" to data from healthy individuals to estimate a no-effect level for sensitive subpopulations, the available data suggest that the magnitude of the safety factor could be relatively small, a factor of two or three at most, as described below.

Data presented in this chapter suggest that 2 and 5 ppm might represent no-observed-effect levels (NOELs) for sensitive and healthy populations, respectively. On the basis of the work of Stevens et al. (1992), who showed that a 1.8-ppm HCl exposure to young asthmatic adults for 45 min, including 15 min of exercise, was without effect, 2 ppm can represent a NOEL for sensitive individuals for a 45-min exposure. Opinions based on general occupational experiences suggest that slight symptoms in adult workers might occur at exposure levels around 5 ppm. Heyroth (1963) and Sayers et al. (1934) suggested that HCl exposures at 1-5 ppm might be detected or cause slight symptoms; Heyroth (1963) and Elkins (1959) indicated that 5-10 ppm is immediately irritating and disagreeable.

Table D-9 outlines mild, moderate, and severe effects that might be anticipated following HCl exposure, according to the descriptors established in Chapter 4.[1] The concentrations shown in Table D-9 at which

---

[1] Mild effects are reversible within 48 hr and do not interfere with normal activity or require medical attention. Moderate effects are irreversible effects that do not alter organ function or interfere with normal activity, or they are reversible effects that alter organ function or interfere with normal activity.

(Continued on next page)

TABLE D-9 Anticipated Health Effects Following HCl Exposure in Healthy Humans for Up to 1 Hr[a]

Severity	Concentration, ppm	Effects
Mild effects	≥5	Eye and nasal irritation, irritation of the throat, slight cough, headache; no significant pathological changes anticipated
Moderate effects	≥20	Frequent coughs, eye and nasal burning, shortness of breath, flulike symptoms; mild inflammatory changes might occur in upper respiratory tract
Severe effects	≥100	Difficulty breathing, chest pain, burning throat, disorientation, corneal opacity; significant ulceration, erosion, and inflammatory changes might occur in upper respiratory tract; inflammatory changes including pulmonary edema might occur in lower respiratory tract

[a]The concentrations listed are the lowest at which effects in the specified severity category might occur in some members of a healthy population. As exposure concentrations increase, more individuals are expected to be affected and the severity of response within an individual is expected to increase. For exposures of less than 1 hr, the concentrations at which mild, moderate, and severe effects might begin to occur in a healthy population could be somewhat higher than those listed. How much higher depends on the relationship between exposure duration and concentration to the effects seen. The concentrations shown in the table are based on available human data. Because of the limitations associated with these data, Haber's law should not be used for extrapolations, especially for those at the higher concentrations shown in the table. That relationship is described in Chapter 6.

mild, moderate, and severe effects might begin to occur in some members of a healthy population are derived from industrial hygiene experience and human-response information published by Matt (1889), Henderson and Haggard (1943), Heyroth (1963), Fine et al. (1987), Stevens et al. (1992), and ACGIH (1991). The majority of those data were collected from healthy working individuals. The effects column in Table D-9 includes signs and symptoms reported following human exposures or those reasonably anticipated to occur in humans on the basis of animal studies. The database on human exposures to HCl is weak because much of it depends on opinion rather than documented exposure-re-

---

Persons experiencing moderate effects are likely to seek medical attention. Severe effects are irreversible effects that alter organ function or interfere with normal activities. Severe effects usually require medical attention.

sponse studies. While that type of experiential information is valuable and has been used in establishing OELs, it is difficult to extrapolate to nonoccupational settings and to the general public. The paucity of quantitative human data makes it difficult to evaluate the health effects of exposure to high concentrations of HCl or to develop guidelines for short-term exposure limits based strictly on data derived from human exposures to HCl. Although the effects listed in Table D-9 are classified according to expected severity, it must be emphasized that predicting such severities is based on the subcommittee's best judgment given available data. The subcommittee emphasizes that individuals can vary greatly in their sensitivity to any chemical, such as HCl, particularly at high exposure concentrations.

RESEARCH NEEDS

The data base for assessing the effects of HCl on the respiratory tract at low concentrations is small and much of it is not well documented. Although more modern inhalation toxicity data using animal models would be useful, the critical data that are needed can be provided only by carefully controlled human exposures at low HCl exposure concentrations, particularly between 2 and 20 ppm. Inclusion of asthmatic individuals in the study population is critical if the responses of sensitive individuals are to be understood well.

REFERENCES

ACGIH (American Conference of Governmental Industrial Hygienists). 1991. Hydrogen chloride. Pp. 773-774 in Documentation of the Threshold Limit Values and Biological Exposure Indices, Vol. 2, 6th Ed. American Conference of Governmental Industrial Hygienists, Cincinnati, Ohio.

Albert, R.E., A.R. Sellakumar, S. Laskin, M. Kuschner, N. Nelson, and C. Sayder. 1982. Gaseous formaldehyde and hydrogen chloride induction of nasal cancer in rats. J. Natl. Cancer Inst. 68:597-601.

Anderson, R.C. and Y. Alarie. 1980. Acute lethal effects of polyvinylchloride thermal decomposition products in normal and canulated mice. Toxicologist, p. A3.

Barrow, C.S., Y. Alarie, J.C. Warrick, and M.F. Stock. 1977. Comparison of the sensory irritation response in mice to chlorine and hydrogen chloride. Arch. Environ. Health 32:68-76.

Barrow, C.S., H. Lucia, and Y.C. Alarie. 1979. A comparison of the acute inhalation toxicity of hydrogen chloride versus the thermal decomposition products of polyvinylchloride. J. Combust. Toxicol. 6:3-12.

Bennett, R.R. 1996. Toxicity of HCl and NO_x and Their Concentrations in Launch Ground Clouds. Paper presented to the National Research Council Subcommittee on Rocket Emission Toxicants, Oct. 8, 1996, Irvine, Calif.

Boulet, L.P. 1988. Increases in airway responsiveness following acute exposure to respiratory irritants. Chest 94:476-481.

Boyce, S.H. and K.A. Simpson. 1996. Hydrochloric acid inhalation: Who needs admission? J. Accid. Emerg. Med. 13:422-424.

Buckley, L.A., X.Z. Jiang, R.A. James, K.T. Morgan, and C.S. Barrow. 1984. Respiratory tract lesions induced by sensory irritants at the RD50 concentration. Toxicol. Appl. Pharmacol. 74:417-429.

Burleigh-Flayer, H., K.L. Wong, and Y. Alarie. 1985. Evaluation of the pulmonary effects of HCl using CO_2 challenges in guinea pigs. Fundam. Appl. Toxicol. 5:978-985.

Cohen, M., J.R. Strange, and T. Rothman. 1982. Short-Term Intermittent Exposure to Hydrogen Chloride (Gas and Mist). Final Report. AD-A165 079. Prepared by Enviro Control Division, Dynamac Corp., Rockville, Md., Contract No. DAMD17-79-C-9125, Subtask 10, for the U.S. Army Medical Research and Development Command, Fort Detrick, Frederick, Md.

Crane, C.R., D.C. Sanders, B.R. Endecott, and J.K. Abbott. 1985. Inhalation Toxicology: IV. Times to Incapacitation and Death for Rats Exposed Continuously to Atmospheric Hydrogen Chloride Gas. FAA Rep. FAA-AM-85-4. Federal Aviation Administration, Washington, D.C.

Darmer, K.I., Jr., E.R. Kinkead, and L.C. DiPasquale. 1974. Acute toxicity in rats and mice exposed to hydrogen chloride gas and aerosols. Am. Ind. Hyg. Assoc. J. 35:623-631.

DiPasquale, L.C. and H.V. Davis. 1971. The acute toxicity of brief exposures to hydrogen fluoride, hydrogen chloride, nitrogen dioxide, and hydrogen cyanide singly and in combination with carbon monoxide. Pp. 279-289 in Proceedings of the Second Annual Conference on Environmental Toxicity. AMRL-TR-71-120. Aerospace Medical Research Laboratory, Wright-Patterson Air Force Base, Dayton, Ohio.

Dyer, R.F., and V.H. Esch. 1976. Polyvinyl chloride toxicity in fires: Hydrogen chloride toxicity in fire fighters. JAMA 235:393-397.

Elkins, H.B. 1959. P. 79 in The Chemistry of Industrial Toxicology. New York: John Wiley & Sons.

Fine, A., J.E. Carlyle, and E. Bourke. 1977. The effects of administrations of HCl, NH_4Cl, and NH_4HCO_3 on the excretion of urea and ammonium in man. Eur. J. Clin. Invest. 7:587-589.

Fine, J.M., T. Gordon, J.E. Thompson, and D. Sheppard. 1987. The role of titratable acidity in acid aerosol induced bronchoconstriction. Am. Rev.

Respir. Dis. 135:826-830.

GEOMET Technologies. 1981. Hydrogen Chloride: Report 4, Occupational Hazard Assessment. NIOSH Contract 210-79-0001. U.S. Department of Health and Human Services, National Institute for Occupational Safety and Health, Cincinnati, Ohio. Available from NTIS, Springfield, Va., Doc. No. PB83-105296.

Hartzell, G.E., H.W. Stacy, W.G. Switzer, D.N. Priest, and S.C. Packham. 1985a. Modeling of toxicological effects of fire gases: IV. Intoxication of rats by carbon monoxide in the presence of an irritant. J. Fire Sci. 3:263-279.

Hartzell, G.E., S.C. Packham, A.F. Grand, and W.G. Switzer. 1985b. Modeling of toxicological effects of fire gases: III. Quantification of post-exposure lethality of rats from exposure to HCl atmospheres. J. Fire Sci. 3:195-207.

Hazardous Substances Data Bank. 1996. Hydrochloric Acid. Update 6/8/94. HSBD No. 545. National Library of Medicine, Toxicology Information Program, Bethesda, Md.

Henderson, Y., and H.W. Haggard. 1943. Characteristics of irritant gases. Pp. 126-127 in Noxious Gases and the Principles of Respiration Influencing Their Action. 2nd Rev. Ed. New York: Van Nostrand Reinhold.

Heyroth, F.F. 1963. Halogens. Pp. 831-857 in Toxicology, D.W. Fassett and D.D. Irish, eds., Vol. 2 of Industrial Hygiene and Toxicology, 2nd Ed., F.A. Patty, ed. New York: Interscience.

Higgins, E.A., V. Fiorca, A.A. Thomas, and H.V. Davis. 1972. Acute toxicity of brief exposures to HF, HCl, NO_2, and HCN with and without CO. Fire Technol. 8:120-130.

Hisham, M.W.M., and T.V. Bommaraju. 1995. Hydrogen chloride. Pp. 894-925 in Kirk-Othmer Encyclopedia of Chemical Technology, Vol. 13, 4th Ed., J.I. Kroschwitz and M. Howe-Grant, eds. New York: John Wiley & Sons.

IARC (International Agency for Research on Cancer). 1992. Occupational Exposures to Mists and Vapours from Strong Inorganic Acids; and Other Industrial Chemicals. IARC Monographs on the Evaluation of Carcinogenic Risks to Humans, Vol. 54. Lyon, France: International Agency for Research on Cancer.

Kamrin, M.A. 1992. Workshop on the health effects of HCl in ambient air. Regul. Toxicol. Pharmacol. 15:73-82.

Kaplan, H.L. 1987. Effects of irritant gases on the avoidance/escape performance and respiratory response of the baboon. Toxicology 47:165-179.

Kaplan, H.L., A. Grand, W.R. Rogers, W.G. Switzer, and G.E. Hartzell. 1984. A Research Study of the Assessment of Escape Impairment by Irritant Combustion Gases in Postcrash Aircraft Fires. AD-A146-484. Prepared by Southwest Research Institute, San Antonio, Tex. for the Federal Aviation Administration, Atlantic City Airport, N.J.

Kaplan, H.L., A. Anzueto, W.G. Switzer, and R.K. Hinderer. 1988. Effects of hydrogen chloride on respiratory response and pulmonary function of the baboon. J. Toxicol. Environ. Health 23:473-493.

Kilburn, K. 1996. Effects of a hydrochloric acid spill on neurobehavioral and pulmonary function. J. Environ. Med. 38:1018-1025.

Kirsch, H. and P. Drabke. 1982. Assessing the biological effects of hydrogen chloride [in German]. Z. Gesamte Hyg. 28:107-109.

Kolesar, G.B., S.D. Crofoot, G.J. Sibert, and W.H. Siddigui. 1993. A comparison of the acute inhalation toxicity of methyltrichlorosilane and gaseous hydrogen chloride in the rat [abstract 520]. Toxicologist 13:151.

Kotchen, T.A., K.E. Krzyzaniak, J.E. Anderson, C.B. Ernst, J.H. Galla, and R.G. Luke. 1980. Inhibition of renin secretion by HCl is related to chloride in both dog and rat. Am. J. Physiol. 239:F44-F49.

Lucia, H.L., C.S. Barrow, M.F. Stock, and Y. Alarie. 1977. A semi-quantitative method for assessing anatomic damage sustained by the upper respiratory tract of the laboratory mouse, *Mus musculis*. J. Combust. Toxicol. 4:472-486.

MacEwen, J.D., and E.H. Vernot. 1974. The determination of a 60-minute LC50 for hydrogen chloride in rodents. Pp. 124-128 in Toxic Hazards Research Unit Annual Technical Report 1974. AMRL-TR-74-78. Aerospace Medical Research Laboratory, Wright-Patterson Air Force Base, Dayton, Ohio.

Machle, W., K.V. Kitzmiller, E.W. Scott, and J.F. Treon. 1942. The effect of inhalation of hydrogen chloride. J. Ind. Hyg. Toxicol. 24:222-225.

Malek, D.E., and Y. Alarie. 1989. Ergometer within a whole-body plethysmograph to evaluate performance of guinea pigs under toxic atmospheres. Toxicol. Appl. Pharmacol. 101:340-355.

Matt, L. 1889. Doctoral dissertation [in German]. Julius Maximilians University, Wurzburg, Germany.

NIOSH (National Institute for Occupational Safety and Health). 1994. Documentation for Immediately Dangerous to Life or Health Concentrations (IDLHs). U.S. Department of Health and Human Services, National Institute for Occupational Safety and Health, Division of Standards Development and Technology Transfer, Cincinnati, Ohio. Available from NTIS, Springfield, Va., Doc. No. PB94-195047.

NRC (National Research Council). 1987. Emergency and Continuous Exposure Guidance Levels for Selected Airborne Contaminants. Ammonia, Hydrogen Chloride, Lithium Bromide, and Toluene, Vol. 7. Washington, D.C.: National Academy Press.

NRC (National Research Council). 1991. Permissible Exposure Levels and Emergency Exposure Guidance Levels for Selected Airborne Contaminants. Washington, D.C.: National Academy Press.

Pavlova, T.E. 1976. Disturbance in the development of the progeny of rats exposed to hydrogen chloride [in Russian]. Biull. Eksp. Biol. Med. 82:866-868.

Pellett, G.L., D.I. Sebacher, R.J. Bendura, and D.E. Wornom. 1983. HCl in rocket exhaust clouds: Atmospheric dispersion, acid aerosol characteristics, and acid rain deposition. J. Air Pollut. Control Assoc. 33:304-311.

Perry, W.G., F.A. Smith, and M.B. Kent. 1994. The halogens. Pp. 4487-4490 in Patty's Industrial Hygiene and Toxicology, Vol. 2, Part F, 4th Rev. Ed., G.D. Clayton and F.E. Clayton, eds. New York: John Wiley & Sons.

Remijn, B., P. Koster, D. Houthuijs, J. Boleij, H. Willems, B. Brunekreef, K. Biersteker, C. van Loveren. 1982. Zinc chloride, zinc oxide, hydrochloric acid exposure and dental erosion in a zinc galvanizing plant in the Netherlands. Ann. Occup. Hyg. 25:299-307.

Sayers, R.R., J.M. Dalla Valle, and W.P. Yant. 1934. Industrial hygiene and sanitation surveys in chemical establishments. Ind. Eng. Chem. 26:1251-1255.

Sebacher, D.I., R.J. Bendura, and D.E. Wornom. 1980. Hydrochloric acid aerosol and gaseous hydrogen chloride partitioning in a cloud contaminated by solid rocket exhaust. Atmos. Environ. 14:543-547.

Sellakumar, A.R., C.A. Snyder, J.J. Solomon, and R.E. Albert. 1985. Carcinogenicity of formaldehyde and hydrogen chloride in rats. Toxicol. Appl. Pharmacol. 81:401-406.

Spengler, J.D., M. Brauer, and P. Koutrakis. 1990. Acid air and health. Environ. Sci. Technol. 24:946-956.

Stavert, D.M., D.C. Archuleta, M.J. Behr, and B.E. Lehnert. 1991. Relative acute toxicities of hydrogen fluoride, hydrogen chloride, and hydrogen bromide in nose- and pseudo-mouth-breathing rats. Fundam. Appl. Toxicol. 16:636-655.

Stevens, B., J.Q. Koenig, V. Rebolledo, Q.S. Hanley, and D.S. Covert. 1992. Respiratory effects from the inhalation of hydrogen chloride in young adult asthmatics. J. Occup. Med. 34:923-929.

Symonds, R.B., W.I. Rose, and M.H. Reed. 1988. Contribution of Cl⁻ and Fl⁻-bearing gases to the atmosphere by volcanoes. Nature 334:415-148.

Tarlo, S.M. and I. Broder. 1989. Irritant-induced occupational asthma. Chest 96:297-300.

Toxigenics. 1984. 90-Day Inhalation Toxicity Study of Hydrogen Chloride Gas in B6C3F1 Mice, Sprague-Dawley Rats, and Fischer-344 Rats. Toxigenics, Decatur, Ill.

U.S. Department of Labor. 1998. Occupational Safety and Health Standards. Air Contaminants. Title 29, Code of Federal Regulations, Part 1910, Section 1910.1000. Washington, D.C.: U.S. Government Printing Office.

Wohlslagel, J., L. DiPasquale, and E. Vernot. 1976. Toxicity of solid rocket motor exhaust: Effects of HCl, HF, and alumina on rodents. J. Combust. Toxicol. 3:61-69.

Appendix E

ACUTE TOXICITY OF NITROGEN DIOXIDE

BACKGROUND INFORMATION

HUMAN and animal data indicate that exposure to nitrogen dioxide (NO_2) can produce a variety of toxicological responses of varying degrees of severity depending on the concentration and duration of exposure and on the sensitivity of the population being exposed. Because NO_2 is a gas, the primary route of exposure is via inhalation, making the lung the primary target organ; however, extrapulmonary effects also have been reported.

There have been numerous reviews on the toxicity of NO_2 (NRC 1977; WHO 1977; EPA 1982, 1993). Most have focused on the health effects associated with exposures to low concentrations of NO_2, such as those that might occur in the environment or in the workplace. Relatively few studies focused on toxicological responses following short-term exposures to high concentrations of NO_2.

PHYSICAL AND CHEMICAL PROPERTIES

CAS No.: 10102-44-0
Molecular weight: 46.0
Specific gravity: 1.448 at 20°
Boiling point: 21.15°C
Melting point: -9.3°C
Freezing point: 15°F

Vapor pressure:	720 mm Hg at 20°C
Vapor density:	1.58 (air = 1)
Flash point:	Not applicable
Explosive limit:	Not applicable
Solubility:	Soluble in concentrated nitric and sulfuric acids; decomposes in water; reacts with water forming nitric oxide and nitric acid.
Color:	Reddish brown gas
Conversion factor:	1 ppm = 1.88 mg/m^3 at 20°C 1 mg/m^3 = 0.53 ppm at 20°C

SOURCES AND OCCURRENCE

In the ambient atmosphere, the major sources of NO_2 are the combustion of fossil fuels and motor-vehicle emissions. Indoor sources include such appliances as gas stoves, water heaters, and kerosene space heaters. In the workplace, exposures to NO_2 have been reported in such occupations as electroplating, acetylene welding, agriculture, space exploration, detonation of explosives, certain military activities, and burning of nitrogen-containing propellants (Mohsenin 1994). In such situations, exposure concentrations can be very high. For example, in armored vehicles during live-fire tests, peak concentrations of NO_2 have been measured at over 2,000 parts per million (ppm). That decreases to about 500 ppm after 1 min and decreases to about 20 ppm within 5 min (Mayorga 1994).

Of concern to the Air Force is the presence of NO_x/HNO_3 emissions from rockets that use liquid propellants composed of nitrogen-based compounds. For normal launches, the nitrogen-associated emissions at ground level are negligible. However, in the case of a catastrophic abort, large quantities of nitrogen tetroxide can be released. That gas is rapidly converted to NO_2 and HNO_3, possibly resulting in production of quantities of NO_x/HNO_3 as high as 200,000 lb (see Appendix A).

PHARMACOKINETICS AND METABOLISM

When inhaled, NO_2 reacts with the moisture in the respiratory tract, resulting in the formation of nitric acid (HNO_3). The nitric acid dissociates into nitrates and nitrites. At low concentrations, NO_2 reacts with moisture in the upper respiratory tract, but as the exposure concentration increases, that reaction penetrates into the lower respiratory tract. An increasing respiratory rate, such as might result from exercise, also results in higher concentrations of NO_2 and its products reaching deeper areas of the lung.

Once inhaled, NO_2, or its chemical derivatives, can either remain within the lung or be transported to extrapulmonary sites via the bloodstream, where it can react with hemoglobin to form methemoglobin (MetHb). That reaction has important health implications because MetHb is an ineffective oxygen carrier. Transformation of hemoglobin to MetHb can increase health risks to vulnerable individuals who have hypoxia associated with pulmonary and cardiac disease. Increased levels of nitrates have been reported in the blood and urine following exposure to NO_2, indicating that NO_2 reacts to produce nitrates (EPA 1993).

SUMMARY OF TOXICITY INFORMATION

In this section, the available data on the toxicity of NO_2 to humans and animals are described.

EFFECTS IN HUMANS

Data on the qualitative and quantitative toxicity of NO_2 in humans come from reports of accidental exposures, clinical studies, and epidemiological studies, as described below.

Accidental Exposures

Accidental exposures to NO_2 have been reported in agriculture (150-2,000 ppm), mining explosions (500 ppm), space exploration (250 ppm), military activities (500 ppm), and the burning of nitrogen containing propellants (Mohsenin 1994). NO_2 has an acrid, ammonia-like odor that is irritating and suffocating to heavily exposed individuals. Such accidental-exposure data, together with relevant animal studies, are most useful in establishing emergency short-term exposure limits.

NO_2 can produce a variety of clinical responses, depending on the intensity and duration of the exposure (Lowry and Schuman 1956; Jones et al. 1973). For the most severely exposed, death can occur immediately or be delayed (Mohsenin 1994). Exposure above 150 ppm for 30 min to an hour results in fatal pulmonary edema or asphyxia and can result in rapid death (Lowry and Schuman 1956; NRC 1977; Mayorga 1994). Exposure to NO_2 at concentrations of 150-300 ppm can result in bronchiolitis fibrosa obliterans accompanied by restrictive and obstructive ventilatory defects that might lead to death in 2 to 3 weeks (Lowry and Schuman 1956; NRC 1977; Mayorga 1994). Such exposures would likely produce permanent injury in those surviving the exposure. The LC_{50} (the lethal concentration for 50% of those exposed) for a 1-hr exposure for humans has been estimated to be 174 ppm (Book 1982). Four farmers who entered a freshly filled silo were exposed to high concentrations of NO_2, estimated to range from 200 to 4,000 ppm. Two of the individuals died, and the others experienced immediate cough, dyspnea, and fever, which disappeared after several days but reappeared after about 3 weeks (Lowry and Schuman 1956; EPA 1982). Information on lethality from accidental exposures to NO_2 is summarized in Table E-1A.

At lower exposure concentrations, a variety of nonlethal effects have been observed (see Table E-1B). From 50 to 100 ppm for a 30-min exposure, pulmonary edema and bronchiolitis with focal pneumonitis are likely to develop and last from 6 to 8 weeks; recovery is often spontaneous. Individuals exposed for 30 min at concentrations between 25 and 75 ppm might develop bronchial pneumonia, acute bronchitis, dyspnea, cyanosis, chess pain, rales, headaches, eye irritation, a dry nonproductive cough, and vomiting. Such effects usually are resolved in hours but sometimes are followed by a relapse with shortness of breath, cough, cyanosis, and fever. In addition to its effect on the lung, NO_2 can transform hemoglobin to MetHb (Lowry and Schuman 1956; Grayson 1956; Stern 1968; Milne 1969; EPA 1993). Welders exposed to NO_2 at 3.9 to 5.4 ppm exhibited 2.3% to 2.6% MetHb in their blood (Patty 1963).

In accidental exposures, accurate measurement of exposure concentrations are generally not available. However, during a manned spaceflight, three astronauts were exposed to NO_2 at concentrations reported to be 250 ppm for about 5 min; the peak was at 750 ppm (Hatton et al. 1977; Table E-1B). They reported immediate breathing difficulties that

TABLE E-1A Summary of NO$_2$ Toxicity in Humans: Mortality from Accidental Exposures

Condition	Exposure Duration	Exposure Concentration, ppm	Effect Concentration, ppm	End Points	References
Healthy	Minutes	200-4000	—	2/4 died	Lowry and Schuman 1956
Healthy	30 min	>500	>500	Death in less than 2 d due to pulmonary edema	Lowry and Schuman 1956; Grayson 1956
		>300-400	>300	Fatal edema, bronchopneumonia	Lowry and Schuman 1956; Grayson 1956
		>150-200	>150	Bronchiolitis fibrosa obliterans with death in 3-5 wk	Lowry and Schuman 1956; Grayson 1956
		50-100	50	Bronchiolitis and focal pneumonia with spontaneous recovery	Lowry and Schuman 1956; Grayson 1956
Healthy	1 hr	174	—	LC$_{50}$	Book 1982

TABLE E-1B Summary of NO$_2$ Toxicity in Humans: Nonlethal Effects from Accidental Exposures

Condition	Exposure Duration	Exposure Concentration, ppm	Effect Concentration, ppm	End Points	References
Healthy	5 min	250 with peaks to 750	250 with peaks to 750	Chemical pneumonitis; 4.2% increase in MetHb	Hatton et al. 1977
Healthy (welders)	Daily	3.9-5.4	3.9-5.4	2.3% and 2.6% MetHg in the blood	Patty 1963

Abbreviation: MetHb, methemoglobin.

became more severe within the first 24 hr, and chest radiographs suggested that they suffered diffuse chemical pneumonitis. The MetHb level also increased (4.2%). Several days later, the individuals became asymptomatic (Hatton et al. 1977). Because the exposure was not lethal and recovery was rapid, the exposure concentrations of NO_2 might have been overestimated.

Human Clinical Studies

Human clinical studies of NO_2 exposure have been conducted using healthy subjects and volunteer patients with existing pulmonary disease. Although such controlled exposures offer the best data to directly relate cause and effect in humans, few such studies have been conducted. Because the safety of volunteer subjects is of paramount importance, high exposure concentrations cannot be used, and only a few nonevasive end points usually are measured.

Normal Subjects Some significant responses, which could be attributed to inhalation of NO_2, have been reported at concentrations of more than 1.0 ppm in normal subjects, as described below.

Sensory effects. Concentrations of 13.0 ppm or more resulted in complaints of eye and nasal irritation (Stern 1968). Humans can detect the odor of NO_2 at low concentrations. At 0.12 ppm, 3 of 9 subjects perceived the odor immediately, and 8 of 13 detected concentrations of 0.22 ppm (Henschler et al. 1960). At a higher concentration (0.42 ppm), 8 of 8 subjects recognized the odor (Henschler et al. 1960). Feldman (1974) reported that 26 of 28 subjects had a perception of NO_2 odor at concentrations of 0.11 ppm. Bylin et al. (1985) reported an odor threshold of 0.04 ppm for healthy subjects and 0.08 ppm for asthmatic subjects. However, in another study, exposed subjects were unable to detect the odor at 0.1 ppm (Hazucha et al. 1983). A 5-min exposure to NO_2 at 25 ppm caused slight-to-moderate nasal discomfort in 5 of 7 volunteers and chest pain in 3 of the 7 (Meldrum 1992). Threshold values for impairment of dark adaptation was reported to be 0.07 ppm after 5 min inhalation of NO_2 by mouth or after 25 min inhalation through the nose only (4 of 4 subjects) (Shalamberidze 1967). However, Bondareva (1963) found no evidence of impairment of dark adaptation. Sensory effects in humans exposed to NO_2 for a 0.5 hr or less are summarized in Table E-1C.

TABLE E-1c Summary of NO$_2$ Toxicity in Humans: Sensory Effects

Condition	Exposure Duration	Exposure Concentration, ppm	Effect Concentration, ppm	End Points	References
Olfactory					
Healthy	Minutes	≥13	≥13	Complaints of eye and nasal irritation	Stern 1968
Healthy	Immediate	0.42 0.22 0.12	0.42 0.22 0.12	Perception of odor (8/8) Perception of odor (8/13) Perception of odor (3/9)	Henschler et al. 1960
Healthy	Immediate	0.11	0.11	Perception of odor (26/28)	Feldman 1974
Healthy	Immediate	0.04 0.08	0.04 0.08	Odor threshold for normal and asthmatic subjects	Bylin et al. 1985
Healthy	Immediate	0.1	—	Odor not detected	Hazucha et al. 1983
Healthy	5 min	25.0	25.0	Slight nasal discomfort (5/7) and chest pain (3/7)	Meldrum 1992
Visual					
Healthy	5 min, 25 min	0.07	0.07	Impaired dark adaptation	Shalamberidze 1967

Effects on lung function. von Nieding and Wagner (1977) and von Nieding et al. (1979) reported that healthy subjects exposed to NO_2 for 2 hr at a concentration of 5.0 ppm exhibited increased airway resistance and impaired oxygen exchange in the lung. They also reported a decrease in carbon dioxide diffusion capacity following a 15-min exposure at 5.0 ppm. Other investigators measured increases in airway resistance following a 10-min exposure at 0.7 to 2.0 ppm or at 4 to 5 ppm (Suzuki and Ishikawa 1965; Abe 1967). However, Linn et al. (1985b) and Mohsenin (1988) failed to find any changes in airway resistance or spirometry at concentrations of 4.0 ppm for 75 min or 2.0 ppm for 2 hr. Another investigator found increases in airway resistance in some subjects after a 10- to 120-min exposure to NO_2 at 7.0 ppm, but other individuals tolerated 16 ppm without any such effect (Yokoyama 1972). A 10-min exposure at 4 to 5 ppm resulted in a 40% decrease in lung compliance 30 min after exposure ended (Abe 1967). Healthy subjects exposed at 2.5 and 7.5 ppm for 2 hr had increased airway resistance, but 1.0 ppm did not elicit any such effect (Beil and Ulmer 1976).

Below 1.0 ppm, short-term exposures (2 hr or less) do not appear to cause adverse effects in healthy subjects, at least as indicated by traditional measurement of pulmonary function (Kagawa and Tsuru 1979; Kerr et al. 1979; Toyama et al. 1981; Hazucha et al. 1982; Bylin et al. 1985; Koenig et al. 1985, 1987, 1988; Kagawa 1986; Adams et al. 1987; Drechsler-Parks 1987; Mohsenin 1988; Samet and Utell 1990; Kim et al. 1991). Some investigators reported subtle effects, but those findings are rare and do not reveal any consistent pattern of response (Kulle 1982; Rehn et al. 1982; EPA 1993).

Physiological changes in airway responsiveness to NO_2 have been studied using a variety of stimuli to challenge the airways. With an acetylcholine challenge, a 2-hr exposure to NO_2 at 7.5 ppm, but not at 5.0, 2.5, or 1.0 ppm, resulted in an increase in airway responsiveness to NO_2 (Beil and Ulmer 1976). However, Mohsenin (1988) reported increased airway reactivity to methacholine following a 1-hr exposure to NO_2 at 2.0 ppm.

Table E-1D summarizes the data from clinical studies of human lung function following exposure to NO_2 for 2 hr or less.

Lung biochemical measures in BAL fluid — Markers of pulmonary effects. A number of studies examined the bronchoalveolar lavage (BAL) fluid from humans in an attempt to identify cellular and biochemical responses to NO_2 exposure. No significant changes occurred in the levels of total protein, albumin, or α-2-macroglobulin in BAL fluid taken from healthy volunteers exposed for 3 hr at 0.05 ppm, including three 15-min peak exposures at 2.0 ppm, or exposed for 3 hr continuously at 0.6 or 1.5 ppm without peaks (Frampton et al. 1989; Utell et al. 1991). Individuals exposed to NO_2 at 3 to 4 ppm for 3 hr had a decrease in activity of α-1-protease inhibitor. This inhibitor is important in protecting the lung from proteolytic damage. Mohsenin and Gee (1987) and Mohsenin (1991) suggested that such a reduction would be most significant in individuals with α-1-antitrypsin deficiency. Table E-1E summarizes the data on BAL-fluid markers of pulmonary effects in humans exposed to NO_2 for 2 hr or less.

Host defense mechanisms. The BAL fluid isolated from exercising individuals exposed to NO_2 at 2.0 ppm for 240 min showed an increase in polymorphonuclear neutrophils (PMNs) and a decrease in the phagocytic activity of alveolar macrophages (Devlin et al. 1992). However, Sandstroem et al. (1990) exposed exercising individuals to NO_2 at 4.0 ppm for 20 min on alternate days for 12 days and found enhanced phagocytic activity, a reduction in total cell count, and a decrease in number of mast cells, T and B lymphocytes, and natural killer cells in BAL fluid 24 hr post-exposure. A simple 20-min exposure at 2.25, 4.0, and 5.5 ppm resulted in a different response. The number of mast cells in BAL fluid increased at all exposure concentrations and the number of lymphocytes increased at 4.0 and 5.5 ppm 24 hr post-exposure (Sandstroem et al. 1989). Frampton et al. (1989) exposed humans to NO_2 for 3 hr at 0.6 ppm and reported a reduced ability of macrophages to inactivate the influenza virus.

Because of the effects observed on the alveolar macrophages, other studies have looked for possible consequences of those macrophage changes with other end points, such as increases in respiratory infections and decreases in pulmonary clearance. However, human data examining the effects of NO_2 on normal pulmonary clearance are inconclusive. Although the clearance of soot particles was significantly slower following acute exposure at 5.0 ppm (Schlipköter and Brockhaus 1963), a later study by Rehn et al. (1982) failed to find any significant changes in clearance of radiolabeled Teflon aerosols following 1 hr exposures to NO_2 at 0.3 or 1.0 ppm.

Table E-1F summarizes the data on the effects of NO_2 exposure for 3 hr or less on pulmonary defenses against infection in humans.

Extrapulmonary effects. Extrapulmonary effects have been reported in humans following NO_2 exposure. Chaney et al. (1981) observed increases in blood glutathione levels in exercising humans exposed at

TABLE E-1D Summary of NO_2 Toxicity in Healthy Humans: Pulmonary Function

Condition	Exposure Duration	Exposure Concentration ppm	Effect Concentration, ppm	End Points	References
Healthy	2 hr	5.0	5.0	Increased airway resistance; impaired oxygen exchange	von Nieding and Wagner 1977; von Nieding et al. 1979
Healthy	2 hr	1.0, 2.5, 7.5	≥2.5	Increased airway resistance	Beil and Ulmer 1976
Healthy	2 hr	1.0, 2.5, 5.0, 7.5	7.5	Increased airway responsiveness to acetylcholine	Beil and Ulmer 1976
Healthy	75 min	4.0	—	No change in airway resistance	Linn et al. 1985b
Healthy	2 hr	2.0	—	No change in airway resistance	Mohsenin 1988
Healthy	1 hr	2.0	2.0	Increased airway responsiveness to methalcholine	Mohsenin 1988
Healthy	10 min	0.7-2.0	0.7	Increased airway resistance; effect increased with dose	Suzuki and Ishikowa 1965
Healthy	15 min	5.0	5.0	Decreased CO diffusion capacity	von Nieding and Wagner 1977, von Nieding et al. 1979
Healthy	10-120 min	7.0, 16.0	7.0	Increased airway resistance in some subjects at 7.0 ppm, but some had no effect at 16.0 ppm	Yokoyama 1972
Healthy	10 min	4-5	4-5	40% decrease in lung compliance and increase in airway resistance	Abe 1967

| Healthy | ≤2 hr | <1 | — | No measured adverse effects in healthy subjects | Kagawa and Tsuru 1979; Kerr et al. 1979; Toyama et al. 1981; Hazucha et al. 1982; Bylin et al. 1985; Koenig et al. 1985, 1987, 1988; Kagawa 1986; Adams et al. 1987; Drechsler-Parks 1987; Mohsenin 1988; Samet and Utell 1990; Kim et al. 1991 |

TABLE E-1E Summary of NO_2 Toxicity in Humans: Lung Biochemical Measures in BAL Fluid

Condition	Exposure Duration	Exposure Concentration, ppm	Effect Concentration, ppm	End Points	References
Healthy	3 hr	0.05 with three 15-min peaks at 2.0 or at 0.6 or 1.5 ppm without peaks	—	No change in BAL fluid composition	Utell et al. 1991; Frampton et al. 1989
Healthy	3 hr	3-4	3-4	Decrease in protease inhibitor	Mohsenin and Gee 1987; Mohsenin 1991

Abbreviations: BAL, bronchoalveolar lavage; MetHb, methemoglobin.

TABLE E-1F Summary of NO$_2$ Toxicity in Humans: Host Defenses

Species	Exposure Duration	Exposure Concentration, ppm	Effect Concentration, ppm	End Points	References
Humans	3 hr	0.6	0.6	Reduced ability of macrophages to inactivate influenza virus	Frampton et al. 1989
Humans (exercising)	240 min	2.0	2.0	Increase in number of PMNs in BAL; decrease in phagocytic activity of exposed macrophages	Devlin et al. 1992
Humans	1 hr	5.0	5.0	Slower clearance of soot particles from lung	Schlipköter and Brockhaus 1963
Humans	1 hr	0.3	1.0	No change in nasal or tracheobronchial clearance	Rehn et al. 1982
Humans (exercising)	20 min on alternate days for 12 d	4.0	4.0	Total cell counts reduced; increase in macrophage phagocytic activity; decrease in number of T and B lymphocytes, mast cells, and natural killer cells 24 hr post-exposure	Sandstroem et al. 1990
Humans (exercising)	20 min	2.25, 4.0, 5.5	2.25	Increase in mast cells in BAL fluid at all concentrations; increase in number of lymphocytes at 4.0 and 5.5 ppm 24 hr post-exposure	Sandstroem et al. 1989

Abbreviations: PMNs, polymorphonuclear neutrophils; BAL, bronchoalveolar lavage.

0.2 ppm for 2 hr, but because the effect was small and no other effects were observed in several other blood measurements (e.g., methemoglobin, red-blood-cell (RBC) glutathion (GSH) reductase, immunoglobulins, and complement C3), the authors thought that those responses might have been due to exercise and not to NO_2 exposure. Small but significant decreases in blood pressure in exercising individuals have been reported following exposure to NO_2 at 4.0 ppm for 75 min (Linn and Hackney 1983). A significant increase in plasma histamine was observed in human volunteers exposed four times at 0.3 ppm for 15 min (Kagawa 1986). Table E-1G summarizes the studies of the extrapulmonary effects of NO_2 exposure on healthy humans for 2 hr or less.

Sensitive Subjects Clinical studies have examined the effects of NO_2 exposure on sensitive subjects, because they might be more responsive and affected by lower concentrations of NO_2, which might exacerbate existing disease. Such studies have sought to determine if NO_2 increases airway responsiveness in subjects with asthma or chronic obstructive pulmonary disease (COPD).

Airway hyper-responsiveness to a wide variety of chemical and physical stimuli occurs with asthma. In clinical studies using asthmatic subjects, most significant responses have been associated with short-term (1 to 3 hr) exposures to NO_2 and low concentrations ranging from 0.2 to 0.5 ppm (EPA 1993; see Table E-1D). Those effects are not seen at higher concentrations (i.e., up to 4.0 ppm) (Orehek et al. 1976; EPA 1993). That indicates that the observed effects fail to follow a normal concentration-response relationship. Other investigators have confirmed that finding. Avol et al. (1988) reported an increase in bronchial reactivity to cold air in individuals exposed at 0.3 ppm, but not at 0.6 ppm, following a 2-hr exposure. Evidence indicates that such effects are reversible. Bauer et al. (1986) exposed asthmatic subjects to NO_2 at 0.3 ppm for 20 min at rest, followed by 10 min of exercise, and found that all subjects had an increased response to cold-air bronchoprovocation, but that effect was not present 60 min post-exposure. Mohsenin (1987) found significant increases in airway responsiveness to methacholine in asthmatic subjects following a 1-hr exposure to NO_2 at 0.5 ppm. Orehek et al. (1976) found increased responsiveness in asthmatic subjects to carbachol following a 1-hr exposure at 0.1 ppm. Exposure to NO_2 for 1 hr at 0.4 ppm can potentiate specific airway response of patients with mild asthma to inhaled house-dust mite allergen. No significant effect was observed after similar exposure at 0.1 ppm (Tunnicliffe et al. 1994).

TABLE E-1G Summary of NO_2 Toxicity in Humans: Extrapulmonary Effects

Condition	Exposure Duration	Exposure Concentration, ppm	Effect Concentration, ppm	End Points	References
Healthy (exercising)	2 hr	0.2	0.2	Increase in blood glutathione levels (probably not significant)	Chaney et al. 1981
Healthy	75 min	4.0	4.0	Small but significant increase in blood pressure	Linn and Hackney 1983
Healthy	15 min × 4	0.3	0.3	Increased plasma histamine levels	Kagawa 1986
Healthy (welders)	—	3.9-5.4	3.9-5.4	2.3% and 2.6% MetHb in blood of welders	Patty 1963

Abbreviations: MetHb, methemoglobin.

Others, however, have failed to find either increases in responsiveness or any pulmonary functional changes in asthmatic subjects from exposures ranging from 0.1 to 0.6 ppm for 30 to 120 min (Kerr et al. 1979; Kulle 1982; Hazucha et al. 1982, 1983; Ahmed et al. 1983a,b; Koenig et al. 1985, 1987; Roger et al. 1990; Rubenstein et al. 1990). Even at higher exposure concentrations and longer durations, subjects with mild asthma exposed at 3.0 ppm, with exercise, for 60 min or at 0.3 ppm for 3.75 hr failed to exhibit changes in pulmonary function, symptoms, or increased airway responsiveness to carbachol (Linn et al. 1986; Morrow and Utell 1989).

It is difficult to understand the differences in responses seen in asthmatic subjects exposed to NO_2 at concentrations of a few parts per million or less. The increase in airway responsiveness to various bronchoconstrictors has been observed in some individuals in some studies, and in other studies, the effect was observed only at NO_2 concentrations ranging from 0.2 to 0.5 ppm and was absent at higher concentrations (Avol et al. 1988). Such differences in response both between and within laboratories might be due to differences in the characteristics or severity of the disease from one test group to another or due to the season of the year when the studies were conducted. In many of the studies, the exposures were accompanied by exercise; exercise alone can be an important covariate in such studies.

Another potentially susceptible group that has been studied is individuals with COPD, such as emphysema and chronic bronchitis. In subjects with chronic bronchitis, exposure for 15 min to NO_2 decreased blood PaO_2 at 4 to 5 ppm and increased airway resistance at concentrations of 1.6 ppm or more (von Nieding et al. 1979). Exposure to NO_2 for 15 min at concentrations between 1.6 and 5.0 ppm also caused significant increases in airway resistance in patients with chronic bronchitis, but below 1.5 ppm, no significant changes were observed (von Nieding et al. 1970). Linn et al. (1985a) found no changes in forced vital capacity (FVC) or forced expiratory volume at 1 sec (FEV_1) at concentrations of 0.5, 1.0, or 2.0 ppm in individuals with chronic bronchitis following a 1-hr exposure, although there was evidence of a possible decrease in peak air flow at 2.0 ppm. Morrow and Utell (1989) examined the response of patients with COPD exposed to NO_2 at 0.3 ppm for 3.75 hr and reported only small decreases in FVC and FEV_1 with mild exercise. It is not obvious why some studies report that individuals with COPD experience pulmonary effects with exposure to NO_2 at a few parts per million and others do not. However, COPD patients might experience some pulmonary functional changes following brief high exposures to NO_2. However, in the asthmatic and COPD populations, the effects from the interaction of the disease state and NO_2 exposure remain questionable.

Table E-1H summarizes the data from clinical studies of the responses of asthmatic and bronchitic subjects to NO_2.

Epidemiological Studies

Most community studies are concerned primarily with effects resulting from low environmental exposure concentrations of NO_2. Such studies have not been able to clearly document the health risks for humans exposed to ambient levels of NO_2. This section will not review all of these studies, but refers the reader to EPA's (1993) Air Quality Criteria for Oxides of Nitrogen, which provides a comprehensive review of all the existing NO_2 epidemiological studies.

Most epidemiological studies that have examined populations for adverse responses to NO_2 have looked at either changes in normal lung function or increases in respiratory illness, especially in children. Although some studies suggest a possible association between NO_2 exposure and an increase in respiratory disease in children, the concentrations of NO_2 in such environments were usually very low (0.1 ppm or less) (Shy et al. 1970a,b; Pearlman et al. 1971; Melia et al. 1977; Speizer et al. 1980; Love et al. 1982). Other investigators have not been able to repeat those findings (Florey et al. 1979; Keller et al. 1979; Melia et al. 1982). The difference in findings has led to the conclusion that if an effect exists, it is subtle and difficult to distinguish from other environmental effects (EPA 1993). A similar conclusion has been drawn from those epidemiological studies examining the effects of NO_2 on pulmonary function (EPA 1993). Because of the low exposure concentrations of NO_2, the extended exposure durations, and the presence of other toxic chemicals in the air, evidence from epidemiological studies is of little value for establishing short-term exposure limits for accidental releases of NO_2.

EFFECTS IN ANIMALS

Numerous health effects from exposure to NO_2 have been confirmed in several species of animals. It is likely that such effects could occur in humans if appropriate exposures were encountered.

TABLE E-1H Summary of NO$_2$ Toxicity in Sensitive Humans: Pulmonary Function

Condition	Exposure Duration	Exposure Concentration, ppm	Effect Concentration, ppm	End Points	References
Asthma	30 min (10-min exercise)	0.3	0.3	Significantly increased bronchial reactivity to cold air	Bauer et al. 1986
Asthma	1 hr	0.5	0.5	Increased airway responsiveness to methacholine	Mohsenin 1987
Asthma	1 hr	0.1	0.1	Increased airway reactivity to carbachol (13/20)	Orehek et al. 1976
Asthma	1 hr	0.1, 0.4	0.4	Increased specific airway response to inhaled house-dust mite allergens	Tunnicliffe et al. 1994
Asthma	1 hr 3.75 hr	3.0 0.3	— —	No changes in pulmonary function; nonresponsive to carbachol	Morrow and Utell 1989; Linn et al. 1986
Asthma	2 hr	0.3, 0.6	0.3	Increased bronchial reactivity to cold at 0.3 but not at 0.6	Avol et al. 1988
Asthma	75 min (exercise)	0.15, 0.30, 0.60	—	No changes in pulmonary function, symptoms, or airway responsiveness to methacholine	Roger et al. 1990
Chronic bronchitis	15 min	1-8	4-5	Reduced alveolar partial pressure of oxygen at 4-5 ppm (arterialized capillary blood); airway resistance increased at ≥1.6 ppm but not at 1.0 ppm	von Nieding et al. 1979
Chronic bronchitis	15 min	0.5, 1.5, 1.6, 5.0	1.6	Significant increase in airway resistance at ≥1.6 but not at lower concentrations; decrease in earlobe blood PO$_2$ at 5.0 ppm, probably starting at 4 ppm	von Nieding et al. 1970

Mortality

The lethal concentration of NO_2 varies from species to species and depends on the duration of exposure. Book (1982) reported LC_{50} values for a 1-hr exposure to NO_2 at 99 ppm for mice, 110 ppm for rats, 91 ppm for guinea pigs, 140 ppm for rabbits, and 130 ppm for dogs. For shorter exposure times, the LC_{50} for rats was 415 ppm, 201 ppm, and 162 pm for a 5-, 15-, and 30-min exposure, respectively (Book 1982). The LC_{50} for the rabbits exposed for 15 min was 315 ppm (Carson et al. 1962). Those studies also indicate that brief high-concentration exposures to NO_2 are more lethal than longer lower-concentration exposures that result in the same or higher total exposure (i.e., exposure concentration (C) multiplied by exposure duration (T)). Hine et al. (1970, as cited in EPA 1982) estimated a threshold concentration for mortality after a 1-hr exposure to be 40 to 50 ppm for a number of species of animals. Once the threshold concentration is exceeded, the death rate increases as the exposure period is lengthened. At 75 ppm, the LT_{50} (time at which 50% of the test animals die) ranges from 2.3 hr for mice, 2.7 hr for rabbits, 3.5 hr for rats, 4.0 hr for guinea pigs, to more than 8 hr for dogs. The NRC (1985) also cited threshold concentrations for acute mortality of 40 to 50 ppm for 1-hr exposures for several species of animals.

Exercise combined with exposure at high concentrations of NO_2 markedly increases the severity of edematous responses and subsequent mortality in animals. Mortality of exercising rats exposed at 1,000 ppm for 1.5 min was 80% higher than mortality in nonexercising rats exposed at 1,500 ppm for 1 min (Lehnert et al. 1994). Rats exposed for 2 min at 1,000 ppm exhibited 100% mortality following exercise (Lehnert et al. 1994). Three squirrel monkeys exposed for 2 hr at 50 ppm died following exposure (Henry et al. 1969).

Table E-2A summarizes the experimental data on the mortality of animals exposed to NO_2 for 2 hr or less.

Pulmonary Injury

Inhalation of NO_2 produces morphological evidence of pulmonary injury. The extent of the injury is related to the sensitivity of the target cell

TABLE E-2A Summary of NO$_2$ Toxicity in Animals: Mortality

Species	Exposure Duration	Exposure Concentration, ppm	Effect Concentration, ppm	End Points	References
Mouse	1 hr	99	—	LC$_{50}$	Book 1982
Mouse	2.3 hr	75	—	LT$_{50}$	Hine et al. 1970
Rat	1.5 min (exercise)	1,000	—	80% higher mortality with exercise than without exercise	Lehnert et al. 1994
	1.0 min (exercise)	1,500	—		
Rat	2.0 min (exercise)	1000	1,000	100% mortality	Lehnert et al. 1994
Rat	5 min	415	—	LC$_{50}$	Book 1982
	15 min	201	—	LC$_{50}$	
	30 min	162	—	LC$_{50}$	
	1 hr	110	—	LC$_{50}$	
Rat	3.5 hr	75	—	LT$_{50}$	Hine et al. 1970
Guinea pig	4.0 hr	75	—	LT$_{50}$	
Rabbit	2.7 hr	75	—	LT$_{50}$	
Dog	>8 hr	75	—	LT$_{50}$	
Guinea pig	1 hr	91	—	LC$_{50}$	Book 1982
Rabbit	1 hr	140	—	LC$_{50}$	
Dog	1 hr	130	—	LC$_{50}$	
Squirrel monkey (n = 3)	2 hr	50	—	100% mortality	Henry et al. 1969
Rabbit	15 min	315	—	LC$_{50}$	Carson et al. 1962

Abbreviations: LC$_{50}$, concentration at which 50% of the test animals die (for a specified exposure duration); LT$_{50}$, time at which 50% of the test animals die (for a given exposure concentration).

or tissue and the dose of NO_2 delivered to the site. Once inhaled, NO_2 affects mainly the bronchioles and adjacent alveolar spaces, where it can produce edema. Although a 5-min exposure of rats at 25 ppm did not produce any histopathological changes, exposure at higher concentrations (50, 75, 100 ppm) did produce mild lung injury, including type II hyperplasia and the appearance of pulmonary alveolar fibrin (Lehnert et al. 1994). Those effects progressed with increasing NO_2 concentrations (150, 200, 250 ppm). As exposure time increased from 5 to 15 and 30 min, the level of type II hyperplasia correlated with increased exposure concentration, and alveolar fibrin appeared at concentrations of 25, 50, 75 and 100 ppm. The fibrin response increased with increasing exposure concentration (Lehnert et al. 1994). Those studies indicate that brief exposures to high concentrations of NO_2 (e.g., 5 min at 50 ppm) are more hazardous than longer exposures to lower concentrations (e.g., 30 min at 25 ppm) producing the same or higher C × T product. A similar C × T relationship was reported with lower concentrations and longer exposures (Gardner et al. 1979).

Histopathological examination of sheep exposed to NO_2 by tracheal tube at 500 ppm for 15 to 20 min revealed patchy exudative material in all lung lobes and an increase in PMNs and mononuclear leukocytes (Januszkiewicz et al. 1992; Januszkiewicz and Mayorga 1994). When the concentration was reduced to 100 ppm for 15 min, only a modest increase in number of leukocytes was found compared with the increase found at 500 ppm (Januszkiewicz et al. 1992; Januszkiewicz and Mayorga 1994). Rats exposed to NO_2 delivered through a sealed face for 15 min at 100 ppm exhibited a significant increase in edema and associated pathological lesions, whereas rats exposed at 25 or 50 ppm did not (Stavert and Lehnert 1990).

A series of studies reported the response of rats at high concentrations of NO_2, ranging from 25 to 250 ppm for 1 to 30 min. A significant increase in lung wet weight (LWW) resulted from a single 5- and 15-min exposure at 150, 200, or 250 ppm but not at 25, 50, 75 or 100 ppm (Lehnert et al. 1994). A single 2-min exposure at 150 ppm also did not result in an increase in LWW (Lehnert et al. 1994). When the exposure duration was increased to 30 min, a significant increase in LWW was observed at 50 ppm (Stavert and Lehnert 1990). All rats exposed to NO_2 for either 15 or 30 min at 200 and 250 ppm ultimately died. Exposure for 1 min to a high burst of NO_2 at concentrations of 500, 1,000, 1,500, and 2,000 ppm all resulted in significant increases in LWW (Lehnert et al. 1994). The percentage change in LWW increased with increasing exposure concentration. Exercise potentiated lung injury in the rats, resulting in further increases in LWW, extent and severity of alveolar fibrin, and red-blood-cell (RBC) extravasation post-exposure at 100 ppm for 15 min (Lehnert et al. 1994). LWWs measured in rats 25 hr post-exposure to NO_2 either at 100 ppm for 15 or 30 min, at 300 ppm for 5 min, or at 1,000 ppm for 1 or 2 min significantly increased over LWWs in control rats (Lehnert et al. 1994).

When dogs were exposed to NO_2 at 37 ppm for 4 hr, the gross and histological findings were negative (Guidotti and Liebow 1977). However, electron microscopy revealed subtle changes, such as an increase in endothelial redundancy and frequency of vesicle formation and changes in surface-to-volume ratios in capillary endothelial cells (Guidotti 1980). Dogs exposed for 1 hr at concentrations ranging from 3 to 16 ppm gave evidence of pulmonary edema at concentrations of 7.0 ppm or more (Dowell et al. 1971).

Some additional damage to alveolar cell mitochondria and cell membranes at concentrations of 3 ppm or more has been reported in dogs (Dowell et al. 1971). A 4-hr exposure of rats at 0.5 ppm resulted in rupture and loss of cytoplasmic granules in mast cells (Thomas et al. 1967). When the concentration was increased to 1.0 ppm and the exposure time cut to 1 hr, there was degranulation and a decrease in number of mast cells. Those responses were reversible. Cats exposed for 3 hr at 80 ppm showed degeneration of Clara cells and loss of cilia 12 hr post-exposure (Langloss et al. 1977). Clara-cell hyperplasia was evident 48 hr post-exposure. There was edema and neutrophilic emigration and extravasation of RBCs, bronchiolar congestion, increases in number of macrophages, and hyperplasia of type II cells (Langloss et al. 1977).

Table E-2B summarizes the evidence for pulmonary injury in animals following exposure to NO_2 for 4 hr or less.

Effects on Lung Function

Both short-term and long-term exposures to NO_2 produce changes in pulmonary function. Exposures of rats to various concentrations of NO_2 for durations of 1 to 20 min produced changes in minute ventilation, tidal volumes, and breathing frequencies (Lehnert et al. 1994). Minute ventilation was reduced by 7% and 15% in rats exposed at 100 ppm for 15 and 20 min, respectively. A 10-min exposure, however, did not produce any changes. Exposures at higher concentrations and shorter dura-

TABLE E-2B Summary of NO$_2$ Toxicity in Animals: Morphological and Pathological Effects on the Lung

Species	Exposure Duration	Exposure Concentration, ppm	Effect Concentration, ppm	End Points	References
Rat	15 min	200	—	40% increase in LWW	Elsayed et al. 1995
Rat	1 min	500, 1,000, 1,500, 2,000	≥500	Increasing LWW with increasing dose	Lehnert et al. 1994
Rat	15 min	100	100	Exercise increased severity of lung injury over effects seen with no exercise	Lehnert et al. 1994
Rat	2 min	150	—	No increase in LWW	Lehnert et al. 1994
Rat	15 min	25, 50, 100	100	Pulmonary edema and pathological lesions seen only at the highest concentration	Stavert and Lehnert 1990
Rat	30 min	10, 25, 50	≥50	Increase in LWW	Stavert and Lehnert 1990
Rat	5, 15 min	25, 50, 75, 100, 150, 200, 250	≥150	Increase in LWW post-exposure at ≥150 ppm for 5 min; at ≥100 ppm for 15 min	Lehnert et al. 1994
Rat	5 min	25, 50, 75, 100, 150, 200, 250	≥50	Type II hyperplasia and appearance of alveolar fibrin, dose-response evident	Lehnert et al. 1994
Rat	15 min, no exercise	25, 50, 75, 100, 150, 200, 250	25	All exposures resulted in alveolar fibrin; ≥50 ppm produced type II hyperplasia	Lehnert et al. 1994
Rat	30 min	25, 50, 75, 100	≥25	No hyperplasia at 25 ppm, but increase in appearance of alveolar fibrin at all concentrations; exercise potentiated lung injury	Lehnert et al. 1994
Rat	4 hr	0.5	0.5	–Rupture and loss of cytoplasmic granules in most cells (reversible)	Thomas et al. 1967
Rat	1 hr	1.0	1.0	–Degranulation and decrease in number of mast cells (reversible)	

Species	Duration	Concentration	Effects	Reference
Dog	60 min	3-16	≥3.0	Pulmonary edema at ≥7.0 ppm and evidence of cell membrane changes at ≥3.0 ppm	Dowell et al. 1971
Dog	4 hr	37	37	Subtle changes in morphology with EM, alveolar desquamation, pulmonary edema; no gross effects with light microscopy	Guidotti and Liebow 1977; Guidotti 1980
Sheep	15-20 min by nasotracheal intubation	500	500	Patchy exudative material in all lobes; increase in number of PMNs and mononuclear leukocytes	Januszkiewicz and Mayorga 1994
Sheep	15 min by nasotracheal intubation	100, 500	100	Increased number of leukocytes at 100 ppm; at 500 ppm there was patchy lobular exudate and accumulation of leukocytes in alveolar sacs and interalveolar capillaries	Januszkiewicz et al. 1992; Januszkiewicz and Mayorga 1994
Cat	3 hr	80	80	Degeneration and hyperplasia of Clara cells, loss of cilia, edema; increase in number of macrophages and hyperplasia of Type II cells	Langloss et al. 1977
Squirrel monkey	2 hr	10-50	10 15 35 50	Concentration-related effects: —alveolar septa breaks and expanded alveoli; —patchy interstitial infiltration of lymphocytes; —areas of lung collapsed and alveolar septa became basophilic; —frank edema, lungs showing extreme vesicular dilation and collapsed alveoli with lymphocyte infiltration, bronchi showing absence of cilia	Henry et al. 1969

Abbreviations: LWW, lung wet weight; EM, electron microscopy; PMNs, polymorphonuclear neutrophils.

tions (1,000 ppm for 1 and 2 min) resulted in a still greater decrease (i.e., 20% and 28%). The reduction in minute ventilation was due primarily to a reduction in tidal volume, which decreased as much as 40% at the highest concentration tested (1,000 ppm). Breathing frequencies increased only slightly during those exposures (Lehnert et al. 1994). Rats exposed to NO_2 for 15 min at 200 ppm showed a decrease in inspired minute ventilation during exposure (Elsayed et al. 1995).

A biphasic response consisting of an immediate and delayed reaction was reported in sheep exposed to NO_2 by intubation (nasal passages anesthetized by Xylocaine), at 500 ppm for 15 min (Januszkiewicz and Mayorga 1994). The immediate effect is manifested by an increase in minute-ventilation rate (+64%), an increase in respiratory rate (+129%), and a nonsignificant reduction in tidal volume (-20%). About 6 hr later, airway resistance and hypoxemia increased and lung compliance decreased (Januszkiewicz and Mayorga 1994).

When sheep were exposed to NO_2 for 15 min at 100 ppm by intubation, only a modest increase in minute ventilation was found, compared with the increase seen following a similar exposure at 500 ppm (Januszkiewicz et al. 1992). There were no changes in pulmonary resistance and no demonstrable pathological lesions (Januszkiewcz et al. 1992). When NO_2 was delivered to the sheep by face mask, the response was less severe than when delivered directly to the lung, indicating some protective effect afforded by the nasal passage and upper airway (Januszkiewicz and Mayorga 1994).

Abraham et al. (1980) reported that sheep exposed to NO_2 at 7.5 or 15 ppm for 2 or 4 hr showed effects at only the highest concentration and exposure duration (15 ppm for 4 hr); the effects were increases in pulmonary resistance immediately following the exposure.

Other species have been tested for pulmonary functional effects. Guinea pigs exposed for 1 hr at NO_2 concentrations ranging from 7 to 146 ppm showed concentration-related increases in respiratory rate and decreases in tidal volume, as well as an increase in sensitivity to inhaled histamine aerosols (Silbaugh et al. 1981). Exercising dogs exposed for 2 hr at 5 ppm had a statistically significant decrease in the ventilation equivalent for O_2 (Kleinman and Mautz 1991). When squirrel monkeys were exposed for 2 hr at 10 or 14 ppm and challenged after exposure with a bacterial aerosol, tidal volume decreased but returned to normal or increased within 24 hr post-exposure (Henry et al. 1969).

Table E-2c summarizes the morphological and pathological effects on the lungs of animals following exposure to NO_2 for 4 hr or less.

TABLE E-2c Summary of NO$_2$ Toxicity in Animals: Pulmonary Function

Species	Exposure Duration	Exposure Concentration, ppm	Effect Concentration, ppm	End Points	References
Rat	1, 2 min	1,000	1,000	—Minute ventilation and tidal volume reduced by 20% at 1 min and 28% at 2 min	Lehnert et al. 1994
Rat	10, 15, 20 min	100	100	—Minute ventilation reduced by 7% at 15 min and 15% at 20 min	
Rat	15 min	200	200	Decrease in inspired minute-ventilation rate	Elsayed et al. 1995
Guinea pig	1 hr	7-146		Concentration-related increases in respiratory rate; decrease in tidal volume; increase in sensitivity to histamine	Silbaugh et al. 1981
Dog	2 hr (exercise)	5.0	5.0	Decrease in ventilation equivalent for O$_2$	Kleinman and Mautz 1991
Sheep	15 min by intubation	100	100	Modest increase in minute ventilation	Januszkiewicz et al. 1992
Sheep	15 min by intubation	500	500	Increase in minute ventilation; increase in respiration rate; increase in airway resistance; hypoxemia; decrease in compliance	Januszkiewicz and Mayorga 1994
Sheep	2 hr 4 hr	7.5 15	15 (4 hr)	Increase in pulmonary resistance only at 15 ppm for 4 hr	Abraham et al. 1980
Squirrel monkey	2 hr	10, 14 before bacterial aerosol	10	Decrease in tidal volume (reversible)	Henry et al. 1969

Effects on Lung Biochemistry

Biochemical studies of lung lavage fluid recovered from exposed animals have focused on either the mechanism of toxicity or the detection of indicators of NO_2-induced tissue and cell injury. Following exposure of rats to NO_2 at 100 ppm for 15 min, isolated BAL fluid indicated a significant increase in the number of PMNs and lavageable protein but no increase in the number of macrophages (Lehnert et al. 1994). Those effects became evident 8 hr post-exposure and subsided after several hours in clean air. At still higher concentrations (200 ppm), Elsayed et al. (1995) found that a 15-min exposure of rats resulted in a decrease in the number of macrophages, increases in LWW, and an increase in the number of epithelial cells in BAL fluid. In addition, those authors reported a raised lipid peroxidation rate measured as fluorescent materials in isolated lipid extracts.

When sheep were exposed (lung only, nasal intubation under local anaesthesia) at 500 ppm for 15 to 20 min, they had significant increases in protein, albumin, and number of epithelial cells in BAL fluid and a significant decrease in the number of alveolar macrophages in BAL fluid (Januszkiewicz and Mayorga 1994; Mayorga et al. 1995). A similar response has been reported in dogs exposed at 200 ppm for 1 hr (Man et al. 1990).

A 3-hr exposure of guinea pigs at 5.0 ppm resulted in an increase in lipid content of the lavage fluid if the animals were vitamin-C depleted; no increase occurred if they were not vitamin-C depleted (Selgrade et al. 1981).

Total lecithin was reduced in BAL fluid in dogs exposed for 1 hr at 7 to 16 ppm but not at 3 ppm. There was a decrease in total phospholipids in BAL fluid from animals with intra-alveolar edema (Dowell et al. 1971). There was also an increase in the amount of unsaturated fatty acids in the phospholipids. Those changes were not noted in animals exposed at 3 ppm (Dowell et al. 1971).

Products of arachidonic acid metabolism in the lungs are also affected by NO_2. The concentration of thromboxane B_2 was higher in BAL fluid in rabbits exposed at 1.0 ppm for 2 hr (Schlesinger et al. 1990). When the NO_2 concentration was increased to 3 ppm or 10 ppm, the concentration of thromboxane B_2 in BAL fluid was depressed; at 10 ppm, the 6-keto-prostaglandin $F_{1\alpha}$ concentrations in BAL fluid also were depressed.

Table E-2D summarizes the animal studies of biochemical changes in BAL fluid in response to exposure to NO_2 for 3 hr or less.

Host Defense Mechanisms

The host defense system of the lung is one of the systems whose function has been shown to be altered by NO_2 exposure in several species of animals, possibly because NO_2 interferes with the efficiency of clearing unwanted substances from the lung. NO_2 can disrupt the effectiveness of the mucociliary -clearance system. Exposure of sheep at 15 ppm for 2 hr resulted in a slowing of mucus transport (Abraham et al. 1980). No effect was seen at 7.5 ppm. Another study with rabbits exposed at 10 ppm for 2 hr found no effects on bronchial clearance (Schlesinger et al. 1988). However, Vollmuth et al. (1986) reported a concentration-related acceleration in clearance of particles from the lungs of rabbits following a 2-hr exposure at concentrations of 0.3, 1.0, 3.0 and 10 ppm, and the greatest increase occurred at the two lowest concentrations. That effect could possibly be considered an adaptive response to the exposure.

Pulmonary bactericidal activity decreased progressively with increasing concentrations of NO_2. The effect was present in mice exposed for 4 hr at 7.0, 9.2, and 15 ppm, but not at 1.9 or 3.8 ppm (Goldstein et al. 1973). At the highest concentration tested, the bactericidal activity was reduced by 50% (Goldstein et al. 1973). With a 17-hr exposure, that dysfunction occurred at concentrations as low as 2.3 ppm (Goldstein et al. 1973). Exposure of mice for 4 hr at 5 or 10 ppm reduced the lung's bactericidal activity and increased the severity of *Mycoplasma* infection (Parker et al. 1989). Exposure of mice to NO_2 at 5.0 ppm, but not at lower concentrations (0.5, 1.0, and 2.0 ppm), affected lung bactericidal activity against *Mycoplasma* (Davis et al. 1992). A 4-hr exposure of mice at concentrations of 4 ppm or more resulted in a concentration-related decrease in bactericidal activity, but no effect occurred at 2.5 ppm (Jakab 1988). A 2-hr exposure at 10, 15, or 35 ppm resulted in delayed clearance of inhaled bacteria from the lungs of squirrel monkeys (Henry et al. 1969). Those reports are consistent with studies showing that macrophages obtained from rabbits exposed at 10 ppm for 3 hr had a 50% reduction in phagocytic activity (Gardner et al. 1969). Also, a 2-hr exposure at 8 ppm increased the number of PMNs in the BAL fluid of those animals compared with controls (Gardner et al. 1969).

TABLE E-2D Summary of NO_2 Toxicity in Animals: Lung Biochemical Measures in BAL Fluid

Species	Exposure Duration	Exposure Concentration, ppm	Effect Concentration, ppm	End Points	References
Rat	15 min	100	100	Increase in protein concentrations and PMNs in BAL fluid (reversible)	Lehnert et al. 1994
Rat	15 min	200	200	Evidence of increased rate of lipid peroxidation; decrease in number of macrophages, but increase in number of epithelial cells in BAL	Elsayed et al. 1995
Guinea pig (vitamin-C depleted)	3 hr	5.0	5.0	Increase in BAL lipid concentrations	Selgrade et al. 1981
Rabbit	2 hr	1, 3, 10	≥1.0	Increased concentrations of thromboxane B_2 in BAL at 1.0 ppm, but decrease at other exposure concentrations; at 10 ppm, depression of 6-keto-prostaglandin $F_{1\alpha}$ concentrations in BAL	Schlesinger et al. 1990
Dog	1 hr	3, 7, 16	≥7	Decrease in total phospholipids, increase in amount of unsaturated fatty acids, no effect at 3.0	Dowell et al. 1971
Dogs	1 hr	200	200	Increase in protein, albumen, and number of epithelial cells in BAL fluid, but decrease in macrophage number	Man et al. 1990
Sheep	15-20 min by tracheal intubation	500	500	Increase in protein, albumin, and number of epithelial cells in BAL, but decrease in macrophage number	Januszkiewicz and Mayorga 1994; Mayorga et al. 1995

Abbreviations: PMNs, polymorphonuclear neutrophils; BAL, bronchoalveolar lavage.

Other studies have shown that macrophages isolated from rabbits exposed for 3 hr at 25 ppm reduced production of interferon (Valand et al. 1970). A similar exposure at 15 ppm showed that macrophages had a lower capacity to phagocytize and to develop virus-induced resistance (Acton and Myrvik 1972).

Different experimental approaches have been used to determine the functional efficiency of the host's pulmonary defenses following NO_2 exposure. Many studies measured the host's efficiency by challenging the NO_2-exposed animals with a pulmonary infection. A linear exposure-duration-versus-response function was observed in mice exposed at 0.5 to 28 ppm, indicating that mortality increases with length of exposure (Gardner et al. 1979). Mortality also increased with increasing concentrations of NO_2, as indicated by the steeper slopes of the exposure-duration-versus-response function at higher concentrations (Gardner et al. 1979). In general, exposure to high concentrations of NO_2 for brief periods resulted in more severe pulmonary infections and greater mortality than exposure to lower concentrations for longer periods that produced similar C × T products. For example, when the C × T was held constant, exposure for 1.5 hr at 14 ppm (C × T = 21 ppm•min) increased mortality of mice by nearly 60% (Gardner et al. 1977). A 14-hr exposure at 1.5 ppm (C × T = 21 ppm•min) resulted in only a 12% increase in incidence of infection (Gardner et al. 1977). A 3-hr exposure of mice at concentrations of 2 ppm or more, but not at concentrations of 1.5 ppm, resulted in increased infection from the *Streptococcus* organism (Ehrlich 1980). When a *Klebsiella* organism was used, the NO_2 concentrations required to produce an increase in infections following a 2-hr exposure was 3.5 ppm or more, and no effect was seen at 1.5 or 2.5 ppm (Ehrlich 1980). Even when the bacterial infection was given 27 hr following an acute 2-hr exposure at 14 ppm, a significant increase in mortality was still evident (Ehrlich 1980). An increase in pulmonary infections was seen in hamsters and squirrel monkeys following a 2-hr exposure at 35 and 50 ppm, respectively (Ehrlich 1975, 1980).

Table E-2E summarizes the data on the effects of exposures to NO_2 on the pulmonary defenses against infection in animals for 4 hr or less.

Extrapulmonary Effects

Evidence suggests that NO_2 or its reaction products penetrate the lung

TABLE E-2E Summary of NO$_2$ Toxicity in Animals: Host Defenses

Species	Exposure Duration	Exposure Concentration, ppm	Effect Concentration, ppm	End Points	References
Mouse	1.5 hr	14	14	60% increase in induced pulmonary infection	Gardner et al. 1977
Mouse	2 hr	1.5, 2.5, 3.5, 5, 10, 15	≥3.5	Concentration-related increase in induced pulmonary infection with *Klebsiella*	Ehrlich 1980
Mouse	3 hr	1.5, 2.0, 5.0	≥2.0	Concentration-related increase in induced infection with *Streptococcus*	Ehrlich 1980
Mouse	6 min to 12 mo	1.5 to 28	Depends on C and T	Increased induced infectious disease with increased T and C, but concentration more important than T	Gardner et al. 1979
Mouse	4 hr	1.9, 3.8, 7.0, 9.2, 15.0	≥7.0	Bactericidal activity decreased by 7%, 14%, and 50% at three highest concentrations, respectively	Goldstein et al. 1973
Mouse	4 hr	5, 10	5	Reduced bactericidal activity; increased severity of induced *Mycoplasma* infection	Parker et al. 1989
Mouse	4 hr	0.5, 1.0, 2.0, 5.0	5.0	Reduced bactericidal activity	Davis et al. 1992
Mouse	4 hr	2.5, 4.0, 5.0, 10, 15	≥4.0	Concentration-related decrease in bactericidal activity	Jakab 1988
Hamster	2 hr	5.0, 25.0, 35.0	35	Increased incidence of induced pulmonary infection; no effect ≤25 ppm	Ehrlich 1975, 1980
Rabbit	2 hr	0.3, 1.0, 3.0, 10.0	≥0.3	Concentration-related acceleration of pulmonary clearance of particles; greatest effect at lowest concentration	Vollmuth et al. 1986
Rabbit	2 hr	8.0	8.0	Increase in number of PMNs in BAL	Gardner et al. 1969
Rabbit	2 hr	10.0	—	No effect on bronchial-clearance rate	Schlesinger et al. 1988
Rabbit	3 hr	25.0	25.0	Reduction in macrophages' ability to produce interferon	Valand et al. 1970

Rabbit	3 hr	15.0	Reduced phagocytic activity of macrophages and reduced ability to develop virus-induced resistance	Acton and Myrvik 1972
Rabbit	3 hr	10.0	50% reduction in macrophages' phagocytic activity	Gardner et al. 1969
Sheep	2 hr	7.5, 15.0	Effects on mucociliary clearance, slowing of mucus transport	Abraham et al. 1980
Squirrel monkey	2 hr	10, 15, 35	Delayed clearance of inhaled micro-organisms	Henry et al. 1969
Squirrel monkey	2 hr	50	Increase in pulmonary-infection incidence	Ehrlich 1975

Abbreviations: C, concentration; T, time (exposure duration).

and enter the bloodstream, producing a wide array of health effects beyond the lung. Rats exposed for 15 min at 200 ppm had an increase in carboxyhemoglobin (COHb) (Elsayed et al. 1995). Investigators found that when sheep were exposed at 500 ppm (lung only, nasal intubation under local anaesthesia) for 15 to 20 min, both pulmonary arterial pressure and pulmonary artery wedge pressure were significantly higher 24 hr post-exposure, and a small, but significant, increase in blood MetHb was reported (Januszkiewicz and Mayorga 1994; Mayorga et al. 1995). However, when mice were exposed for 1 hr at 5 to 40 ppm, there was no evidence of MetHb, yet increased nitrite and nitrate concentrations were found in the blood (Oda et al. 1981). In contrast, Case et al. (1979) found concentration-related increases in MetHb in mice exposed at 1 to 30 ppm for 18 hr.

Several studies have identified direct effects on the kidney and liver from exposures to NO_2, but the exposures used in those studies usually lasted several days or weeks (EPA 1993). However, Miller et al. (1980) found that exposure of mice at 0.25 ppm for 3 hr resulted in a significant increase in pentobarbital-induced sleeping time. Such a response implies a potential effect on some aspects of liver metabolism. Also, a single 2-hr exposure at 0.3 to 4.0 ppm produced increased levels of ascorbic acid in the liver of mice (Veninga and Lemstra 1975). Information on the effects of NO_2 on the central nervous system (CNS), behavior, and reproduction and developmental effects is limited to a few studies of longer exposure durations; the relation of those effects to humans is uncertain (EPA 1993).

Although exercise has been shown to increase the severity of several of the pulmonary responses, a 15-min exposure to NO_2 at 25, 50, and 100 ppm also reduced the rat's ability to perform maximal exercise as assessed by measuring maximum oxygen consumption (Mayorga et al. 1995). A 1-min exposure at 100 ppm also significantly reduced exercise performance (Mayorga et al. 1995).

Table E-2F summarizes the studies of the extrapulmonary effects of exposures to NO_2 in animals for durations of 2 hr or less.

ESTABLISHED INHALATION EXPOSURE LIMITS

Table E-3 lists existing exposure limits for civilian and military populations. Table E-4 lists Army incapacitation criteria for NO_2. Figure E-1 shows the relation among the civilian exposure limits listed in Table E-3.

TABLE E-2F Summary of NO$_2$ Toxicity in Animals: Extrapulmonary Effects

Species	Exposure Duration	Exposure Concentration, ppm	Effect Concentration, ppm	End Points	References
Mouse	1 hr	5-40	—	No evidence of MetHb, but increased levels of nitrite and nitrate in blood	Oda et al. 1981
Mouse	18 hr	1-30	—	Concentration-related increases in MetHb and decrease in catalase and iron transferrin activity in the blood	Case et al. 1979
Rat	15 min	200	200	Increased COHb	Elsayed et al. 1995
Sheep	15-20 min	500	500	Increase in pulmonary artery and pulmonary artery wedge pressure; small increase in MetHb	Mayorga et al. 1995; Januszkiewicz and Mayorga 1994
Mouse	3 hr	0.25	0.25	Significant increase in pentobarbital-induced sleeping time	Miller et al. 1980
Mouse	2 hr	0.3-4.0	≥0.3	Increased levels of ascorbic acid in liver	Veninga and Lemstra 1975
Rat	15 min	25, 50, 100	≥25	Concentration-related decrease in maximal exercise	Mayorga et al. 1995
Rat	1 min	25, 50, 100	100	Significant reduction in exercise performance	Mayorga et al. 1995

Abbreviations: COHb, carboxyhemoglobin; MetHb, methemoglobin.

TABLE E-3 Currently Recommended Civilian and Military Human Exposure Limits for NO_2

Exposure Limit	Concentration, ppm	Reference
EPA		
NAAQS	0.053	EPA 1971
LOC	2	EPA 1987
ACGIH		
TLV-TWA	3	ACGIH 1991
TLV-STEL	5	ACGIH 1991
NIOSH		
IDLH	20	NIOSH 1994
REL	1 (15-min STEL)	NIOSH 1994
OSHA PEL	5 (ceiling)	U.S. Dept. of Labor 1998
NRC SPEGLs		
1 hr	1.0	NRC 1985
2 hr	0.5	NRC 1985
4 hr	0.25	NRC 1985
8 hr	0.12	NRC 1985
16 hr	0.06	NRC 1985
24 hr	0.04	NRC 1985
AIHA EELs		
5 min	35	AIHA 1964
15 min	25	AIHA 1964
30 min	20	AIHA 1964
60 min	10	AIHA 1964
U.S. Army Acceptable Human Criteria in Armored Vehicle During Live Fire Testing		
15 min	50	Mayorga 1994
5 min	100	Mayorga 1994

Abbreviations: EPA, U.S. Environmental Protection Agency; NAAQS, National Ambient Air Quality Standard; LOC, level of concern; ACGIH, American Conference of Governmental Industrial Hygienists; TLV, Threshold Limit Value; TWA, time-weighted average; STEL, short-term exposure limit; NIOSH, National Institute for Occupational Safety and Health; IDLH, immediately dangerous to life and health; REL, recommended exposure limit; OSHA, Occupational Safety and Health Administration; PEL, permissible exposure level; NRC, National Research Council; SPEGL, short-term public emergency guidance level; AIHA, American Industrial Hygiene Association; EEL, emergency exposure limits.

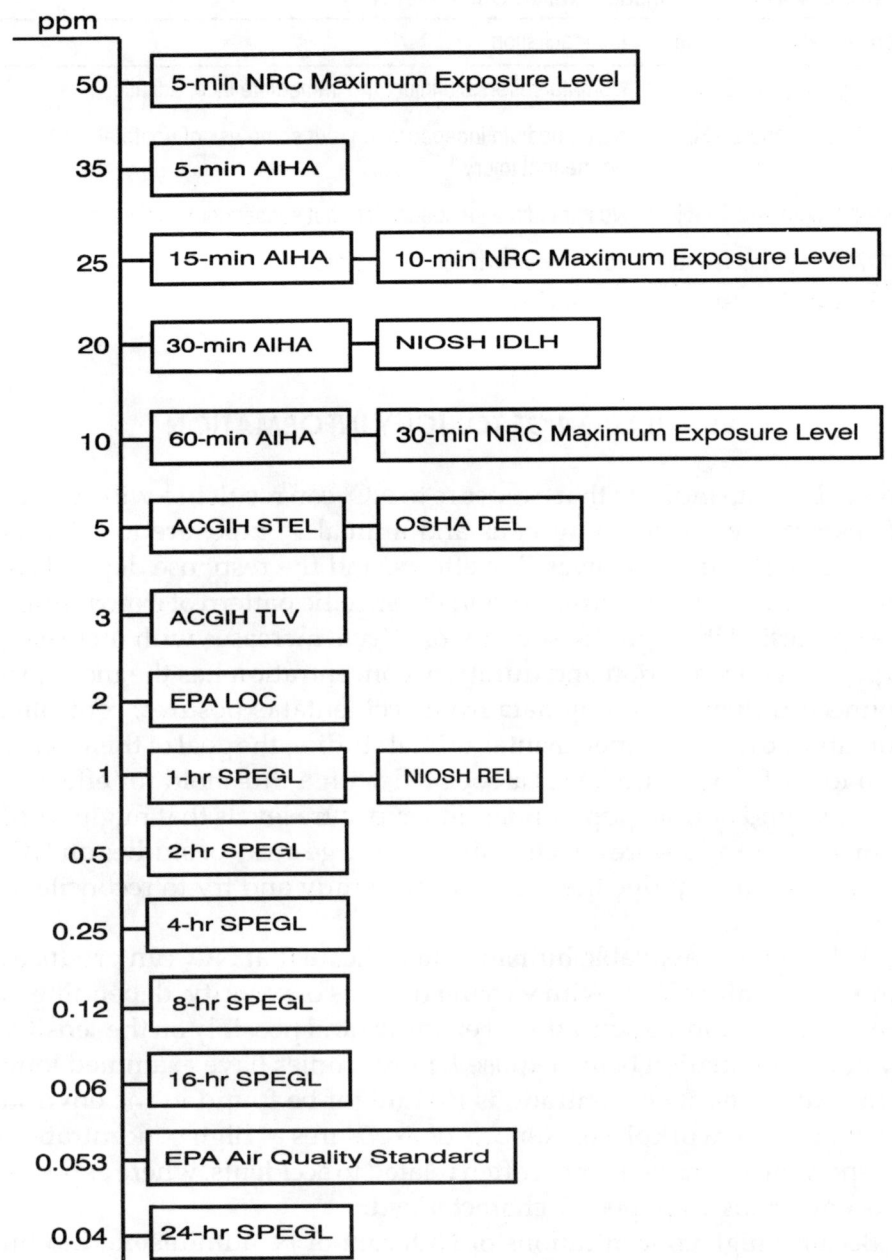

FIGURE E-1 Currently recommended exposure limits for human exposure to NO_2 (see Table E-3 for sources).

TABLE E-4 U.S. Army Incapacitation Criteria for NO_2

Concentration and Time	Incapacitation
1-50 ppm and 1-30 min	Nonfatal reversible injury; no immediate incapacitation
50-100 ppm and 20-30 min	No immediate incapacitation, but some risk of nonfatal permanent injury
150-200 ppm and 30 min	No immediate incapacitation, but subsequent fatal injury
300-750 ppm and few min	100% incapacitation or fatal injury

Source: Adapted from Mayorga 1994.

EVALUATION OF TOXICITY INFORMATION

Available data indicate that exposure to NO_2 can result in a wide variety of respiratory effects in humans and animals. Exposure to NO_2 can cause reversible and irreversible effects, and the response depends on the concentration, the duration, and the specific pattern of exposure and the species. Although the severity of effects increases with increasing exposure concentration and duration, concentration has the more pronounced influence. Using data from accidental exposures, controlled human studies, and experimental animal studies, the goal of this chapter is to identify exposure levels associated with a threshold for effects in sensitive and normal populations and exposure levels that might result in moderate and severe effects. Given the large array of studies on NO_2, it is important to judge the value of each study and try to reconcile divergent results.

Although the available human data indicate that NO_2 can produce a variety of health effects with varying degrees of severity, depending on the concentration and duration of exposure and possibly on the sensitivity of the population being exposed, most studies have examined long-term exposures at concentrations that might be found in the environment or in the workplace. Reports of exposures at high concentrations for short durations were most often related to accidents, where exposure concentrations were poorly characterized.

Because high concentrations of NO_2 cannot be administered to humans, health effects seen in animals must be extrapolated to humans. The effects seen in animals exposed to NO_2 can reasonably be expected to occur in humans if the exposure concentrations were adequate to induce the effect. However, quantitative extrapolation from animals to humans requires quantitative information on interspecies similarities and differences in dosimetry and sensitivity. Some of that type of information is available; however, it is not adequate for quantitative extrapolation. The relation between C × T and health effects for NO_2 exposures is especially important for determining the importance of short-term peak concentrations compared with time-weighted-average (TWA) concentrations over longer exposure durations (e.g., 1 hr or more). Following a rocket launch, high concentrations of NO_2 will most likely exist with other rocket-emission toxicants in the atmosphere. Exposure to NO_2 together with other emission chemicals (although not HCl and HNO_3 for normal launches) might result in additive effects.

Certain groups might be more sensitive to the effects of NO_2 exposure than others; those groups are persons with pre-existing cardiopulmonary problems and children. Lower concentrations of NO_2 might affect those groups more than healthy adults, or the severity of an effect at a given concentration might be greater. The data available to judge the potential impact of NO_2 on particularly sensitive subgroups are not consistent, however. NO_2 is emitted in the home environment by gas cooking and has been reported to increase susceptibility to respiratory-tract infections in young children. However, that effect is believed to result from long-term exposures, which are not applicable to rocket-launch situations. Short-term exposures of human volunteers to NO_2 have generally provided conflicting results. The ATS (1996) compiled a list of nine controlled studies of asthmatic subjects published since 1980. For seven of the studies, no changes in pulmonary function or airway responsiveness were listed. One study (Bauer et al. 1986) showed that exposure of asthmatic subjects to NO_2 at a concentration of 0.3 ppm potentiated exercise-induced bronchospasm and airway hyperactivity after cold-air provocation. By comparison, exposure of healthy humans at concentrations up to 4 ppm usually failed to affect pulmonary function (ATS 1996). However, in another study, no significant lung-function alterations could be found in asthmatic subjects exposed at 0.3 ppm NO_2 for 1 hr (Morrow and Utell 1989). Mohsenin (1987) found heightened airway reactivity in asthmatic subjects exposed to NO_2 at 0.5 ppm for 1 hr. However, Linn et al. (1985b) observed no effects from exposures to NO_2 at concentrations up to 4 ppm for 1.25 hr in individuals with asthma or in healthy individuals; that observation was attributed to potential adaptation of the subjects who lived in an area with frequent increases in common air pollutants. Responsiveness to a 4-hr exposure to NO_2 at 0.3 ppm was slightly greater in patients with chronic obstructive pulmonary disease (COPD) than in elderly healthy subjects; interindividual variation in responsiveness also was substantially greater in elderly subjects than in the other groups (Morrow et al. 1992). Thus, some study comparisons suggest that individuals with asthma or COPD begin respond to NO_2 at concentrations (0.3 ppm) approximately 10-fold lower than do healthy individuals (4 ppm), while other comparisons suggest no difference in the exposure concentration representing a threshold for effect in the two subgroups. Studies have not been conducted using high concentrations of NO_2.

Exposure to NO_2 can produce a variety of clinical response depending on the intensity and duration of exposure. From the data presented in the preceding sections, hazards associated with short-term exposures can be classified into three general levels of response: (1) mild, (2) moderate, or (3) severe, as described in Chapter 4.[1] Table E-5 outlines the subcommittee's assessment of mild, moderate, and severe adverse health effects associated with exposure to NO_2 and the exposure concentrations at which such effects might begin to occur in healthy adults exposed for durations up to 1 hr. As indicated in Table E-1D, numerous studies have failed to identify measurable health effects in healthy subjects exposed at less than 1 ppm for up to 2 hr. At 4 to 5 ppm, Abe (1967) noted a 40% decrease in lung compliance and an increase in airway resistance in healthy humans exposed for 10 min, although Linn et al. (1985b) found no change in airway resistance for exposures at 4 ppm for 75 min. On the basis a review of case reports of individuals exposed to NO_2 in silos, Lowry and Schuman (1956) concluded that exposure to NO_2 at concentrations of 50 ppm for 30 to 60 min could cause bronchiolitis and focal pneumonia, although recovery could occur without medical intervention.

---

[1] Mild effects are reversible with 48 hr and do not interfere with normal activity or require medical attention. Moderate effects are irreversible effects that do not alter organ function or interfere with normal activity, or they are reversible effects that alter organ function or interfere with normal activity. Persons experiencing moderate effects might seek medical attention. Severe effects are irreversible effects that alter organ function or interfere with normal activities. Severe effects usually require medical attention.

TABLE E-5 Subcommittee Assessment of Anticipated Health Effects Following NO_2 Exposure in Healthy Humans for Up to 1 hr[a]

Severity	Concentration, ppm	Effects
Mild	≥1	No immediate incapacitation; symptomatic effects include: transient discomfort; unpleasant odor; respiratory and eye irritation; acute reversible respiratory function effects; minor changes in hematological indexes; reversible histological effects; changes in normal host defense mechanisms.
Moderate	≥4	No immediate incapacitation; respiratory and eye irritation; reversible changes in respiratory function, pulmonary pathology and morphology; biochemical end points in lung.
Severe	≥50	Serious effects requiring medical treatment or hospitalization; progressive respiratory injury, including edema, permanent pulmonary injury, loss of consciousness, and possible death

[a]The concentrations listed are the lowest estimated concentrations at which effects in the specified severity category might occur in some members of the healthy population. As exposure concentration increases, more individuals are expected to be affected, and the severity of response within an individual is expected to increase. For exposures for less than 1 hr, the concentrations at which mild, moderate, and severe effects might begin to occur in the healthy population could be somewhat higher than those listed. How much higher depends on the relationship between exposure duration and concentration to the effects seen. The concentrations shown in the table are based on available human data. Because of the limitations associated with these data, Haber's law should not be used for extrapolations, especially for those at the higher concentrations shown in the table. That relationship is described in Chapter 6.

Although the effects listed in Table E-5 are classified on the basis of their expected severity, the subcommittee must emphasize that predicting severity is based on its best judgment given the available data. Individuals can vary greatly in their susceptibility to the harmful effects of exposure to any chemical such as NO_2. That factor is especially critical with exposures to high concentrations, even for a short exposure time.

RESEARCH NEEDS

For purposes of the LATRA-ERF model, data that would be most useful to the Air Force would be those from controlled human exposures using sufficient concentrations of NO_2 to produce mild and moderate symptoms over durations of a few minutes to an hour. The exposure protocol should be designed to reveal the relation between exposure duration and exposure concentration in producing mild-to-moderate effects. Both sensitive and healthy groups of individuals should be tested. Subjective reports by the individuals tested and clinical symptoms should be documented at each combination of exposure and response. Pulmonary function also should be measured before, during, and after exposures. A minimum sample size of 10 individuals per group is desirable.

Experiments using the same exposure protocols on mice and rats as humans would be useful to identify the degree of difference in sensitivity to NO_2 between laboratory animals and sensitive and healthy humans.

To evaluate the potential for additive effects among the rocket-emission toxicants, exposure of healthy humans to various combinations of HCl, NO_2, and HNO_3 at concentrations expected to occur following a catastrophic abort might be useful. To be safe, the tests could be limited to exposure concentrations expected to produce mild effects only.

Controlled human exposures at high NO_2 exposure concentrations to determine the sensitivity of individuals with cardiopulmonary impairments and that of healthy individuals are not possible. Thus, to fill this data gap, an animal model that might be expected to react similarly to sensitive humans would be needed. The same animal model probably could be used to investigate this data gap for the other rocket-emission toxicants examined in this report.

REFERENCES

Abe, M. 1967. Effects of mixed NO_2-SO_2 gas on human pulmonary functions: Effects of air pollution on the human body. Bull. Tokyo Med. Dent. Univ. 14:415-433.

Abraham, W.M., M. Welker, W. Oliver, Jr., M. Mingle, A.J. Januszkiewicz, A. Wanner, and M.A. Sackner. 1980. Cardiopulmonary effects of short-term nitrogen dioxide exposure in conscious sheep. Environ. Res. 22:61-72.

ACGIH (American Conference of Governmental Industrial Hygienists). 1991. Documentation of the Threshold Limit Values and Biological Exposure Indices, 6th Ed. American Conference of Governmental Industrial Hygienists, Cincinnati, Ohio.

Acton, J.D., and Q.N. Myrvik. 1972. Nitrogen dioxide effects on alveolar macrophages. Arch. Environ. Health 24:48-52.

Adams, W.C., K.A. Brookes, and E.S. Schelegle. 1987. Effects of NO_2 alone and in combination with O_3 on young men and women. J. Appl. Physiol. 62:1698-1704.
Ahmed, T., R. Dougherty, and M.A. Sackner. 1983a. Effect of NO_2 Exposure on Specific Bronchial Reactivity in Subjects with Allergic Bronchial Asthma. Final Report. Contract CR-83/07/BI. General Motors Research Laboratories, Warren, Mich.
Ahmed, T., R. Dougherty, and M.A. Sackner. 1983b. Effect of 0.1 ppm NO_2 on Pulmonary Functions and Non-specific Bronchial Reactivity of Normals and Asthmatics. Final Report. Contract CR-83/11/BI. General Motors Research Laboratories, Warren, Mich.
AIHA (American Industrial Hygiene Association). 1964. Emergency Exposure Limits. Am. Ind. Hyg. Assoc. J. 25:578-586.
ATS (American Thoracic Society). 1996. Health effects of outdoor air pollution. Part 2. Am. J. Respir. Crit. Care Med. 153:477-498.
Avol, E.L., W.S. Linn, R.C. Peng, G. Valencia, D. Little, and J.D. Hackney. 1988. Laboratory study of asthmatic volunteers exposed to nitrogen dioxide and to ambient air pollution. Am. Ind. Hyg. Assoc. J. 49:143-149.
Bauer, M.A., M.J. Utell, P.E. Morrow, D.M. Speers, and F.R. Gibb. 1986. Inhalation of 0.30 ppm nitrogen dioxide potentiates exercise-induced bronchospasm in asthmatics. Am. Rev. Respir. Dis. 134:1203-1208.
Beil, M., and W.T. Ulmer. 1976. Effect of NO_2 in workroom concentrations on respiratory mechanics and bronchial susceptibility to acetylcholine in normal persons [in German]. Int. Arch. Occup. Environ. Health 38:31-44.
Bondareva, E.N. 1963. Hygienic evaluation of low concentrations of nitrogen oxides present in acid. Pp. 98-101 in USSR Literature on Air Pollution and Related Occupational Diseases. A Survey, Vol. 8, B.S. Levine, ed. Publ. TT-63-11570. U.S. Public Health Service, Washington, D.C.
Book, S.A. 1982. Scaling toxicity from laboratory animals to people: An example with nitrogen dioxide. J. Toxicol. Environ. Health 9:719-725.
Bylin, G., T. Lindvall, T. Rehn, and B. Sundin. 1985. Effects of short-term exposure to ambient nitrogen dioxide concentrations on human bronchial reactivity and lung function. Eur. J. Respir. Dis. 66:205-217.
Carson, T.R., M.S. Rosenholtz, F.T. Wilinski, and M.H. Weeks. 1962. The responses of animals inhaling nitrogen dioxide for single, short-term exposures. Am. Ind. Hyg. Assoc. J. 23:457-462.
Case, G.D., J.S. Dixon, and J.C. Schooley. 1979. Interactions of blood metalloproteins with nitrogen oxides and oxidant air pollutants. Environ. Res. 20:43-65.
Chaney, S., W. Blomquist, P. DeWitt, and K. Muller. 1981. Biochemical changes in humans upon exposure to nitrogen dioxide while at rest. Arch. Environ. Health 36:53-58.
Davis, J.K., M.K. Davidson, T.R. Schoeb, and J.R. Lindsey. 1992. Decreased

intrapulmonary killing of *Mycoplasma* pulmonis after short-term exposure to NO_2 is associated with damaged alveolar macrophages. Am. Rev. Respir. Dis. 145(2 Part 1):406-411.

Devlin, R. D. Horstman, S. Becker, T. Gerrity, M. Madden, and H. Koren. 1992. Inflammatory response in humans exposed to 2.0 ppm NO_2 [abstract]. Am. Rev. Respir. Dis. 145:A456.

Dowell, A.R., K.H. Kilburn, and P.C. Pratt. 1971. Short-term exposure to nitrogen dioxide: Effects on pulmonary ultrastructure, compliance, and the surfactant system. Arch. Intern. Med. 128:74-80.

Drechsler-Parks, D.M. 1987. Effect of Nitrogen Dioxide, Ozone, and Peroxyacetyl Nitrate on Metabolic and Pulmonary Function. Res. Rep. 6. Cambridge, Mass.: Health Effects Institute.

Ehrlich, R. 1975. Interaction Between NO_2 Exposure and Respiratory Infection. Scientific Seminar on Automotive Pollutants. EPA/600/9-75/003. U.S. Environmental Protection Agency, Office of Research and Development, Washington, D.C.

Ehrlich, R. 1980. Interaction between environmental pollutants and respiratory infections. Environ. Health Perspect. 35:89-100.

Elsayed, N.M., S. Smith, D. Ebel, N.V. Gorbounov, M.J. Topper, V.E. Eagon, and M.A. Mayorga. 1995. Pulmonary Alterations after Brief, Nose-Only Exposure of Rats to High Levels of Nitrogen Dioxide (Abstract 19-P-6). International Congress of Toxicology VII, July 2-6.

EPA (U.S. Environmental Protection Agency). 1971. National primary and secondary ambient air quality standards. Fed. Regist. 36(April 30):8186-8201.

EPA (U.S. Environmental Protection Agency). 1982. Air Quality Criteria for Oxides of Nitrogen. EPA/600/8-82-026. U.S. Environmental Protection Agency, Office of Health and Environmental Assessment, Environmental Criteria and Assessment Office, Research Triangle Park, N.C. Available from NTIS, Springfield, Va., Doc. No. PB83-131011.

EPA (U.S. Environmental Protection Agency). 1987. Technical Guidance for Hazards Analysis: Emergency Planning for Extremely Hazardous Substances. Prepared in cooperation with the Federal Emergency Management Agency, Washington, D.C., and U.S. Department of Transportation, Washington, D.C. U.S. Environmental Protection Agency, Office of Solid Waste and Emergency Response, Washington, D.C. Available from NTIS, Springfield, Va., Doc. No. PB93-206910.

EPA (U.S. Environmental Protection Agency). 1993. Air Quality Criteria for Oxides of Nitrogen, Vol. 3. EPA/600/8-91/049cF. U.S. Environmental Protection Agency, Office of Research and Development, Washington, D.C.

Feldman, Y.G. 1974. The combined action on a human body of a mixture of the main components of motor vehicle exhaust gases (carbon monoxide, nitrogen dioxide, formaldehyde, and hexane) [in Russian]. Gig. Sanit. 10:7-10.

Florey, C. du V., R.J.W. Melia, S. Chinn, B.D. Goldstein, A.G.F. Brooks, H.H.

John, I.B. Craighead, and X. Webster. 1979. The relation between respiratory illness in primary schoolchildren and the use of gas for cooking: III. Nitrogen dioxide, respiratory illness, and lung infection. Int. J. Epidemiol. 8:347-353.

Frampton, M.W., A.M. Smeglin, N.J. Roberts, Jr., J.N. Finkelstein, P.E. Morrow, and M.J. Utell. 1989. Nitrogen dioxide exposure in vivo and human alveolar macrophage inactivation of influenza virus in vitro. Environ. Res. 48:179-192.

Gardner, D.E., R.S. Holzman, and D.L. Coffin. 1969. Effects of nitrogen dioxide on pulmonary cell population. J. Bacteriol. 98:1041-1043.

Gardner, D.E., F.J. Miller, E.J. Blommer, and D.L. Coffin. 1977. Relationships between nitrogen dioxide concentration time and level of effect using an animal infectivity model. Pp. 513-525 in International Conference on Photochemical Oxidant Pollution and Its Control. Proceedings, Vol. 1, B. Dimitriades, ed. EPA-600/3-77-001a. U.S. Environmental Protection Agency, Environmental Sciences Research Laboratory, Research Triangle Park, N.C. Available from NTIS, Springfield, Va., Doc. No. PB-264232.

Gardner, D.E., F.J. Miller, E.J. Blommer, and D.L. Coffin. 1979. Influence of exposure mode on the toxicity of NO_2. Environ. Health Perspect. 30:23-29.

Goldstein, E., M.C. Eagle, and P.D. Hoeprich. 1973. Effect of nitrogen dioxide on pulmonary bacterial defense mechanisms. Arch. Environ. Health 26:202-204.

Grayson, R.R. 1956. Silage gas poisoning: Nitrogen dioxide pneumonia, a new disease in agricultural workers. Ann. Intern. Med. 45:393-408.

Guidotti, T.L. 1980. Toxic inhalation of nitrogen dioxide: Morphologic and functional changes. Exp. Mol. Pathol. 33:90-103.

Guidotti, T.L., and A.A. Liebow. 1977. Toxic inhalation of NO_2 in canines. In International Conference on Photochemical Oxidant Pollution and Its Control. Proceedings, Vol. 1, B. Dimitriades, ed. EPA-600/3-77-001a. U.S. Environmental Protection Agency, Environmental Sciences Research Laboratory, Research Triangle Park, N.C. Available from NTIS, Springfield, Va., Doc. No. PB-264232.

Hatton, D.V., C.S. Leach, E. Nicogossian, and N. Di Ferrante. 1977. Collagen breakdown and nitrogen dioxide inhalation. Arch. Environ. Health 32:33-36.

Hazucha, M.J., J.F. Ginsberg, W.F. McDonnell, E.D. Haak, Jr., R.L. Pimmel, D.E. House, and P.A. Bromberg. 1982. Changes in bronchial reactivity of asthmatics and normals following exposures to 0.1 ppm NO_2. Pp. 387-400 in Air Pollution by Nitrogen Oxides. Proceedings of the US-Dutch International Symposium, T. Schneider and L. Grant, eds. Studies in Environmental Science 21. Amsterdam: Elsevier Scientific.

Hazucha, M.J., J.F. Ginsberg, W.F. McDonnell, E.D. Haak, Jr., R.L. Pimmel, S.A. Salaam, D.E. House, and P.A. Bromberg. 1983. Effects of 0.1 ppm nitrogen dioxide on airways of normal and asthmatic subjects. J. Appl. Physiol.

Respir. Environ. Exercise Physiol. 54:730-739.
Henry, M.C., R. Ehrlich, and W.H. Blair. 1969. Effect of nitrogen dioxide on resistance of squirrel monkeys to *Klebsiella pneumoniae* infection. Arch. Environ. Health 18:580-587.
Henschler, D., A. Stier, H. Beck, and W. Neumann. 1960. Olfactory threshold of some important irritant gases and effects in man at low concentrations. Arch. Gewerbepath. Gewerbehyg 17:547-570.
Hine, C.H., F.H. Meyers, and R.W. Wright. 1970. Pulmonary changes in animals exposed to nitrogen dioxide, effects of acute exposures. Toxicol. Appl. Pharmacol. 16:201-213.
Jakab, G.J. 1988. Modulation of Pulmonary Defense Mechanisms Against Viral and Bacterial Infections by Acute Exposures to Nitrogen Dioxide. Res. Rep. 20. Cambridge, Mass.: Health Effects Institute.
Januszkiewicz, A.J., and M.A. Mayorga. 1994. Nitrogen dioxide induced acute lung injury to sheep. Toxicology 89:279-300.
Januszkiewicz, A.J., J.R. Snapper, J.W. Sturgis, D.B. Rayburn, K.A. Dodd, Y.Y. Phillips, G.R. Ripple, D.D. Sharpnack, N.M. Coulson, and J.A. Bley. 1992. Pathophysiologic responses of sheep to brief high-level NO_2 exposure. Inhal. Toxicol. 4:359-372.
Jones, G.R., A.T. Proudfoot, and J.I. Hall. 1973. Pulmonary effects of acute exposure to nitrous fumes. Thorax 28:61-65.
Kagawa, J. 1986. Experimental studies on human health effects of aerosol and gaseous pollutants. Pp. 683-697 in Aerosols: Research, Risk Assessment and Control Strategies, Proceedings of the Second U.S.-Dutch International Symposium, S.D. Lee, T. Schneider, L.D. Grant, and P.J. Verkerk, eds. Chelsea, Mich.: Lewis Publishers.
Kagawa, J., and K. Tsuru. 1979. Respiratory effects of 2-hour exposure to ozone and nitrogen dioxide alone and in combination in normal subjects performing intermittent exercise [in Japanese]. Nippon Kyobu Shikkan Gakkai Zasshi 17:765-774.
Keller, M.D., R.R. Lanese, R.I. Mitchell, and R.W. Cote. 1979. Respiratory illness in household using gas and electricity for cooking: II. Symptoms and objective findings. Environ. Res. 19:504-515.
Kerr, H.D., T.J. Kulle, M.L. McIlhany, and P. Swidersky. 1979. Effects of nitrogen dioxide on pulmonary function in human subjects: An environmental chamber study. Environ. Res. 19:392-404.
Kim, S.U., J.Q. Koenig, W.E. Pierson, and Q.S. Hanley. 1991. Acute pulmonary effects of nitrogen dioxide exposure during exercise in competitive athletes. Chest 99:815-819.
Kleinman, M.T., and W.J. Mautz. 1991. The Effects of Exercise on Dose and Dose Distribution of Inhaled Automotive Pollutants. Res. Rep. 45. Cambridge, Mass.: Health Effects Institute.
Koenig, J.Q., D.S. Covert, M.S. Morgan, M. Horike, N. Horike, S.G. Marshall,

and W.E. Pierson. 1985. Acute effects of 0.12 ppm ozone or 0.12 ppm nitrogen dioxide on pulmonary function in healthy and asthmatic adolescents. Am. Rev. Respir. Dis. 132:648-651.
Koenig, J.Q., D.S. Covert, S.G. Marshall, G. van Belle, and W.E. Pierson. 1987. The effects of ozone and nitrogen dioxide on pulmonary function in healthy and in asthmatic adolescents. Am. Rev. Respir. Dis. 136:1152-1157.
Koenig, J.Q., W.E. Pierson, D.S. Covert, S.G. Marshall, M.S. Morgan, and G. van Belle. 1988. The Effects of Ozone and Nitrogen Dioxide on Lung Function in Healthy and Asthmatic Adolescents. Res. Rep. 14. Cambridge, Mass.: Health Effects Institute.
Kulle, T.J. 1982. Effects of nitrogen dioxide on pulmonary function in normal healthy humans and subjects with asthma and chronic bronchitis. Pp. 477-486 in Air Pollution by Nitrogen Oxides. Proceedings of the US-Dutch International Symposium, T. Schneider and L. Grant, eds. Studies in Environmental Science 21. Amsterdam: Elsevier Scientific.
Langloss, J.M., E.A. Hoover, and D.E. Kahn. 1977. Diffuse alveolar damage in cats induced by nitrogen dioxide or feline calicivirus. Am. J. Pathol. 89:637-644.
Lehnert, B.E., D.C. Archuleta, T. Ellis, W.S. Session, N.M. Lehnert, L.R. Gurley, and D.M. Stavert. 1994. Lung injury following exposure of rats to relatively high mass concentrations of nitrogen dioxide. Toxicology 89:239-277.
Linn, W.S., and J.D. Hackney. 1983. Short-term human respiratory effects of nitrogen dioxide: Determination of quantitative dose-response profiles, phase I. Exposure of healthy volunteers to 4 ppm NO_2. Report CRC-APRAC-CAPM-48-83. Atlanta, Ga.: Coordinating Research Council. Available from NTIS, Springfield, Va., Doc. No. PB84-132299.
Linn, W.S., D.A. Shamoo, C.E. Spier, L.M. Valencia, U.T. Anzar, T.G. Venet, E.L. Avol, and J.D. Hackney. 1985a. Controlled exposure of volunteers with chronic obstructive pulmonary disease to nitrogen dioxide. Arch. Environ. Health 40:313-317.
Linn, W.S., J.C. Solomon, S.C. Trim, C.E. Spier, D.A. Shamoo, T.G. Venet, E.L. Avol, and J.D. Hackney. 1985b. Effects of exposure to 4 ppm nitrogen dioxide in healthy and asthmatic volunteers. Arch. Environ. Health 40:234-239.
Linn, W.S., D.A. Shamoo, E.L. Avol, J.D. Whynot, K.R. Anderson, T.G. Venet, and J.D. Hackney. 1986. Dose-response study of asthmatic volunteers exposed to nitrogen dioxide during intermittent exercise. Arch. Environ. Health 41:292-296.
Love, G.J., S.P. Lan, C.M. Shy, and W.B. Riggan. 1982. Acute respiratory illness in families exposed to nitrogen dioxide ambient air pollution in Chattanooga, Tennessee. Arch. Environ. Health 37:75-80.
Lowry, T., and L.M. Schuman. 1956. Silo-filler's disease: A newly recognized syndrome caused by nitrogen dioxide inhalation with a report of six cases. Univ. Minn. Med. Bull. 27:234-238.

Man, S.F.P., D.J. Williams, R.A. Amy, G.C.W. Man, and D.C. Lein. 1990. Sequential changes in canine pulmonary epithelial and endothelial cell functions after nitrogen dioxide. Am. Rev. Respir. Dis. 142:199.

Mayorga, M.A. 1994. Overview of nitrogen dioxide effects on the lung with emphasis on military relevance. Toxicology 89:175-192.

Mayorga, M.A., A.J. Januszkiewicz, and B.E. Lenhert. 1995. Environmental nitrogen dioxide exposure hazards of concern to the U.S. Army. Pp. 323-343 in Fire and Polymers II: Materials and Tests for Hazard Prevention ACS Symposium Series No. 599. G.L. Nelson, ed. Washington, D.C.: American Chemical Society.

Meldrum, M. 1992. Toxicology of substances in relation to major hazards: Nitrogen dioxide [abstract]. British Library Document Center. London: HMSO.

Melia, R.J.W., C. du V. Florey, D.G. Altman, and A.V. Swan. 1977. Association between gas cooking and respiratory disease in children. Br. Med. J. 2:149-152.

Melia, R.J.W., C. du V. Florey, R.W. Morris, B.D. Goldstein, H.H. John, D. Clark, I.B. Craighead, and J.C. Mackinlay. 1982. Childhood respiratory illness and the home environment: II. Association between respiratory illness and nitrogen dioxide, temperature and relative humidity. Int. J. Epidemiol. 11:164-169.

Miller, F.J., J.A. Graham, J.W. Illing, and D.E. Gardner. 1980. Extrapulmonary effects of NO_2 as reflected by pentobarbital-induced sleeping time in mice. Toxicol. Lett. 6:267-274.

Milne, J.E.H. 1969. Nitrogen dioxide inhalation and bronchitis obliterans. A review of the literature and report of a case. J. Occup. Med. 11:538-547.

Mohsenin, V. 1987. Airway responses to nitrogen dioxide in asthmatic subjects. J. Toxicol. Environ. Health 22:371-380.

Mohsenin, V. 1988. Airway responses to 2.0 ppm nitrogen dioxide in normal subjects. Arch. Environ. Health 43:242-246.

Mohsenin, V. 1991. Lipid peroxidation and antielastase activity in the lung under oxidant stress: Role of antioxidant defenses. J. Appl. Physiol. 70:1456-1462.

Mohsenin, V. 1994. Human exposure to oxides of nitrogen at ambient and supra-ambient concentrations. Toxicology 89:301-312.

Mohsenin, V., and J.B.L. Gee. 1987. Acute effect of nitrogen dioxide exposure on the functional activity of alpha-1-protease inhibitor in bronchoalveolar lavage fluid of normal subjects. Am. Rev. Respir. Dis. 136:646-650.

Morrow, P.E., and M.J. Utell. 1989. Responses of Susceptible Subpopulations to Nitrogen Dioxide. Res. Rep. 23. Cambridge, Mass.: Health Effects Institute.

Morrow, P.E., M.J. Utell, M.A. Bauer, A.M. Smeglin, M.W. Frampton, C. Cox, D.M. Speers, and F.R. Gibb. 1992. Pulmonary performance of elderly normal subjects and subjects with chronic obstructive pulmonary disease exposed to 0.3 ppm nitrogen dioxide. Am. Rev. Respir. Dis. 145:291-300.

NIOSH (National Institute for Occupational Safety and Health). 1994. Documentation for Immediately Dangerous to Life or Health Concentrations (IDLHs). U.S. Department of Health and Human Services, National Institute for Occupational Safety and Health, Division of Standards Development and Technology Transfer, Cincinnati, Ohio. Available from NTIS, Springfield, Va., Doc. No. PB94-195047.

NRC (National Research Council). 1977. Nitrogen Oxides. Washington, D.C.: National Academy Press.

NRC (National Research Council). 1985. Pp. 83-95 in Emergency and Continuous Exposure Guidance Levels for Selected Airborne Contaminants; Vol. 4. Washington, D.C.: National Academy Press.

Oda, H., H. Tsubone, A. Suzuki, T. Ichinose, and K. Kubota. 1981. Alterations of nitrite and nitrate concentrations in the blood of mice exposed to nitrogen dioxide. Environ. Res. 25:294-301.

Orehek, J., J.P. Massari, P. Gayrard, C. Grimaud, and J. Charpin. 1976. Effect of short-term, low-level nitrogen dioxide exposure on bronchial sensitivity of asthmatic patients. J. Clin. Invest. 57:301-307.

Parker, R.F., J.K. Davis, G.H. Cassell, H. White, D. Dziedzic, D.K. Blalock R.B. Thorp, and J.W. Simecka. 1989. Short-term exposure to nitrogen dioxide enhances susceptibility to murine respiratory mycoplasmosis and decreases intrapulmonary killing of *Mycoplasma pulmonis*. Am. Rev. Respir. Dis. 140:502-512.

Patty, F.A. 1963. Inorganic compounds of oxygen, nitrogen, and carbon. Pp. 919-923 in Toxicology, D.W. Fassett and D.D. Irish, eds., Vol. 2 of Industrial Hygiene and Toxicology, 2nd Rev. Ed., F.A. Patty, ed. New York: Interscience.

Pearlman, M.E., J.F. Finklea, J.P. Creason, C.M. Shy, M.M. Young, and R.J. Horton. 1971. Nitrogen dioxide and lower respiratory illness. Pediatrics 47:391-398.

Rehn, T., M. Svartengren, K. Philipson, and P. Camner. 1982. Mucociliary transport in the lung and nose and air resistance after exposure to nitrogen dioxide [in Swedish]. Coal-Health Environment Project, Tech. Rep. 40. Vallingby, Sweden: Swedish State Power Board.

Roger, L.J., D.H. Horstman, W. McDonnell, H. Kehrl, P.J. Ives, E. Seal, R. Chapman, and E. Massaro. 1990. Pulmonary function, airway responsiveness, and respiratory symptoms in asthmatics following exercise in NO_2. Toxicol. Ind. Health 6:155-171.

Rubenstein, I., B.G. Bigby, T.F. Resis, and H.A. Boushey, Jr. 1990. Short-term exposure to 0.3 ppm nitrogen dioxide does not potentiate airway responsiveness to sulfur dioxide in asthmatic subjects. Am. Rev. Respir. Dis. 141:381-385.

Samet, J.M., and M.J. Utell. 1990. The risk of nitrogen dioxide: What have we learned from epidemiological and clinical studies? Toxicol. Ind. Health 6:247-262.

Sandstroem, T., B. Kolmodin-Hedman, N. Stjernberg, and M.C. Andersson. 1989. Inflammatory cell response in bronchoalveolar fluid after nitrogen dioxide exposure of healthy subjects [abstract]. Am. Rev. Respir. Dis. 139(Suppl.):A124.

Sandstroem, T., M.C. Andersson, B. Kolmodin-Hedman, N. Stjernberg, and T. Angstrom. 1990. Bronchoalveolar mastocytosis and lymphocytosis after nitrogen dioxide exposure in man: A time-kinetic study. Eur. Respir. J. 3:138-143.

Schlesinger, R.B., K.E. Driscoll, B.D. Naumann, and T.A. Vollmuth. 1988. Particle clearance from the lungs: Assessment of effects due to inhaled irritants. Ann. Occup. Hyg. 32(Suppl. 1):113-123.

Schlesinger, R.B., K.E. Driscoll, A.F. Gunnison, and J.T. Zelikoff. 1990. Pulmonary arachidonic acid metabolism following acute exposures to ozone and nitrogen dioxide. J. Toxicol. Environ. Health 31:275-290.

Schlipköter, H.-W., and A. Brockhaus. 1963. Versuche über den Einfluss gasförmiger Luftverunreingungen auf die Deposition und Elimination inhalierter Stäube. Zentralbl. Bakteriol. Parasitenkd. Infektionskr. Hyg. Abt. 191:339-344.

Selgrade, M.K., M.L. Mole, F.J. Miller, G.E. Hatch, D.E. Gardner, and P.C. Hu. 1981. Effect of NO_2 inhalation and vitamin C deficiency on protein and lipid accumulation in the lung. Environ. Res. 26:422-437.

Shalamberidze, O.P. 1967. Reflex effects of mixtures of sulfur and nitrogen dioxides. Hyg. Sanit. (USSR) 32:10-15.

Shy, C.M., J.P. Creason, M.E. Pearlman, K.E. McClain, F.B. Benson, and M.M. Young. 1970a. The Chattanooga school children study: Effects of community exposure to nitrogen dioxide. I. Methods, description of pollutant exposure, and results of ventilatory function testing. J. Air Pollut. Control Assoc. 20:539-545.

Shy, C.M., J.P. Creason, M.E. Pearlman, K.E. McClain, F.B. Benson, and M.M. Young. 1970b. The Chattanooga school children study: Effects of community exposure to nitrogen dioxide. II. Incidence of acute respiratory illness. J. Air Pollut. Control Assoc. 20:582-588.

Silbaugh, S.A., J.L. Mauderly, and C.A. Macken. 1981. Effects of sulfuric acid and nitrogen dioxide on airway responsiveness of the guinea pig. J. Toxicol. Environ. Health 8:31-45.

Speizer, F.E., B. Ferris, Jr., Y.M.M. Bishop, and J. Spengler. 1980. Respiratory disease rates and pulmonary function in children associated with NO_2 exposure. Am. Rev. Respir. Dis. 121:3-10.

Stavert, D.M., and B.E. Lehnert. 1990. Nitric oxide and nitrogen dioxide as inducers of acute pulmonary injury when inhaled at relatively high concentrations for brief periods. Inhal. Toxicol. 2:53-67.

Stern, A.C., ed. 1968. Pp. 446-609 in Air Pollution, 2nd Ed. Vol. 1: Air Pollution and Its Effects. New York: Academic.

Suzuki, T., and K. Ishikawa. 1965. Pp. 199-221 in Research on the Effects of Smog on the Human Body: Report of the Specialized Study on Prevention of Air Pollution, No. 2 [in Japanese]. Research Coordination Bureau of the Science and Technology Agency, Tokyo, Japan.

Thomas, H.V., P.K. Mueller, and R. Wright. 1967. Response of rat lung mast cells to nitrogen dioxide inhalation. J. Air Pollut. Control Assoc. 17:33-35.

Toyama, T., T. Tsunoda, M. Nakaza, T. Higashi, and T. Nakadate. 1981. Airway response to short-term inhalation of NO_2, O_3 and their mixture in healthy men. Sangyo Igaku 23:285-293.

Tunnicliffe, W.S., P.S. Burge, and J.G. Ayres. 1994. Effect of domestic concentrations of nitrogen dioxide on airway responses to inhaled allergen in asthmatic patients. Lancet 344(8939-9840):1733-1736.

U.S. Department of Labor. 1998. Occupational Safety and Health Standards. Air Contaminants. Title 29, Code of Federal Regulations, Part 1910, Section 1910.1000. Washington, D.C.: U.S. Government Printing Office.

Utell, M., M.W. Frampton, N.J. Roberts, Jr., J.N. Finkelstein, and P.E. Morrow. 1991. Mechanisms of Nitrogen Dioxide Toxicity in Humans [abstract]. Investigators Report. Cambridge, Mass.: Health Effects Institute.

Valand, S.B., J.D. Acton, and Q.N. Myrvik. 1970. Nitrogen dioxide inhibition of viral-induced resistance in alveolar monocytes. Arch. Environ. Health 20:303-309.

Veninga, T., and W. Lemstra. 1975. Extrapulmonary effects of ozone whether in the presence of nitrogen dioxide or not. Int. Arch. Arbeitsmed. 34:209-220.

Vollmuth, T.A., K.E. Driscoll, and R.B. Schlesinger. 1986. Changes in early alveolar particle clearance due to single and repeated nitrogen dioxide exposures in rabbits. J. Toxicol. Environ. Health 19:255-266.

von Nieding, G., H.M. Wagner, H. Krekeler, U. Smidt, and K. Muysers. 1970. Absorption of NO_2 in Low Concentrations in the Respiratory Tract and its Acute Effects on Lung Function and Circulation. Paper No. MB-15G presented at the Second International Clean Air Congress, Washington, D.C., December.

von Nieding, G., and H.M. Wagner. 1977. Experimental studies on the short-term effect of air pollutants on pulmonary function in man: Two-hour exposure to NO_2, O_3, and SO_2 alone and in combination. Pp. 5-8 in the Proceedings of the Fourth International Clean Air Congress, S. Kasuga, N. Suzuki, T. Yamada, G. Kimura, K. Inagaki, and K. Onoe, eds. Japanese Union of Air Pollution Prevention Associations, Tokyo, Japan.

von Nieding, G., H.M. Wagner, H. Krekeler, H. Loellgen, W. Fries, and A.

Beuthan. 1979. Controlled studies of human exposure to single and combined action of NO_2, O_3, and SO_2. Int. Arch. Occup. Environ. Health 43:195-210.

WHO (World Health Organization). 1977. Environmental Health Criteria 4: Oxides of Nitrogen. Geneva, Switzerland: World Health Organization.

Yokoyama, E. 1972. The respiratory effects of exposure to SO_2-NO_2 mixtures on healthy subjects [in Japanese]. Jpn. J. Ind. Health 14:449-454.

Appendix F

ACUTE TOXICITY OF NITRIC ACID

BACKGROUND INFORMATION

NITRIC acid (HNO_3) is a colorless, photochemically stable gas in the atmosphere (EPA 1993). It is highly soluble in water to form an aqueous HNO_3 solution. Fuming HNO_3 is concentrated nitric acid that contains dissolved NO_2. Fuming nitric acid is a yellow-to-red fuming liquid with an acrid, suffocating odor. Because it is so volatile, HNO_3 gas at normal atmospheric concentrations does not condense into an aerosol. However, aerosols of aqueous HNO_3 are readily formed by passing clean air over reagent-grade aqueous HNO_3 (Koenig et al. 1989a). Due to the high aqueous vapor content of rocket-exhaust clouds, HNO_3 would likely exist in the aerosol form inside the clouds.

PHYSICAL AND CHEMICAL PROPERTIES

CAS No.:	7697-37-2
Synonyms:	azotic acid, aqua fortis, hydrogen nitrate (many others)
Molecular weight:	63
Specific gravity:	1.50
Melting pint:	$-42°C$
Boiling point:	$83°C$
Vapor pressure:	47.8 mm Hg at $20°C$
Odor threshold:	0.27 ppm (AIHA 1997)
Conversion factor:	1 ppm = 2.58 mg/m^3 at $25°C$
	0.388 mg/m^3 = 1 ppm at $25°C$

Occurrence and Use

HNO_3 is widely used by a number of industries. In the chemical industry, it is used for the manufacture of metallic nitrates, sulfuric acid, aqua regia, arsenic acid and derivatives, nitrous acid and nitrites, oxalic acid, phthalic acid, and so forth. HNO_3 is used for the manufacture of trinitrophenol, trinitrotoluene, nitroglycerin, and various dyes and pharmaceuticals. Much of the NO and NO_2 emitted to the atmosphere from air-pollution sources is converted to HNO_3. EPA (1993) compiled measurements of average concentrations of HNO_3 in the continental United States; those ranged from 0.5 to 3 µg/m3 for 13 rural sites and from 1.1 to 2.7 µg/m3 for 5 urban sites. A 9-day average concentration of HNO_3 for Claremont, CA was 11 µg/m3 (4.4 ppb) (Wolff et al. 1991). Daily averages can be as high as 60 µg/m^3 (26 ppb) and hourly averages as high as 200 µg/m^3 (80 ppb) (EPA 1982; Lioy and Lippmann 1986; Lippmann 1989a,b). HNO_3 is produced at very low concentrations in rocket emissions from the combustion of hydrazine and N_2O_4 under normal launch conditions but at significant concentrations when a launch is aborted after ignition for rockets using liquid propellants.

Pharmacokinetics and Metabolism

The disposition of HNO_3 is not easily determined. It reacts immediately with respiratory mucous membranes after inhalation and does not appear to be absorbed after oral administration (Gosselin et al. 1984). Instead, it causes erosion of the gastrointestinal (GI) mucosal membranes, which produces severe GI distress. Following inhalation exposure, some HNO_3 might decompose to other nitrogen oxides, which might be absorbed by the bloodstream (EPA 1993) (see Appendix E).

Summary of Toxicity Information

The toxicity of HNO_3 is predominately associated with the extremely corrosive nature of this strong acid. In addition, it is an excellent oxidizing agent and reacts immediately with any tissue to cause such effects as skin burns, eye irritation, coughing, dyspnea, and pulmonary edema. Delayed toxicity, possibly as a result of the decomposition of HNO_3 to other nitrogen oxides, could produce methemoglobinemia, but no documentation exists to support that hypothesis (EPA 1993). Respiratory disorders, including pulmonary edema, can occur several hours after an acute exposure and are probably related to inflammation resulting from cellular necrosis in lung tissues. Alveolar type II cells and cell hyperplasia of alveoli are primary cellular responses in the deep lung in animals treated with HNO_3 by instillation (1% solution). Bronchiolitis and alveolitis are associated with instillation of 1% HNO_3 in rats. There are no data concerning the developmental or reproductive effects of HNO_3 (EPA 1993).

Very little is known about the effects of HNO_3 vapor on animals or humans, and no long-term studies have been reported. An aqueous aerosol of HNO_3 can be generated by passing clean air over reagent-grade aqueous HNO_3 solution. Exposures to this aerosol should approximate the exposures of military and civilian populations to the combustion clouds that are produced by rocket emissions at ground level. Some information is known about the effect of HNO_3 gas on human respiratory function. The reported experimental exposures to HNO_3 as an aerosol or as a gas have been generally for short durations (40 min to 4 hr) that approximate the potential exposure duration for individuals in the vicinity of a launch.

EFFECTS IN HUMANS

There is no doubt that very high exposure concentrations of HNO_3 are lethal to humans. "Rapidly progressive pulmonary edema of delayed onset" was observed after an exposure (10-15 min) of three young healthy men to fumes from an explosion of a tank that contained approximately 1,736 liters (L) of 66% HNO_3 (Hajela et al. 1990). The onset of "respiratory difficulties" occurred approximately 4-6 hr after the accident; all died within 24 hr of the exposure.

In a study with humans, exposure of 12 nonsmoking subjects with mild asthma for 3 min to an "acid fog" that was 30 milliosmolar (mOsm) at pH 2 significantly increased specific airway resistance (Balmes et al. 1989). The approximate concentration of HNO_3 in those studies was very high, 40 mg/m^3 (15 ppm). Subjects inhaled the aerosols through a mouthpiece from an ultrasonic nebulizer. Bronchoconstriction was correlated with acidity of the fog, not the nature of the acid, since fogs made up of either HNO_3 or H_2SO_4 or both showed equally potent effects. These studies showed that very short exposures to high concentrations of HNO_3 can cause moderate-to-severe effects in sensitive humans.

Aris et al. (1993) conducted an excellent study to determine the effects of HNO_3 gas, not aerosol, in healthy humans. They designed the study to reflect the conditions of exposure that might occur in dry weather. The test subjects (eight males and two females) were exposed to HNO_3 at 500 µg/m³ (0.2 ppm) in a 2.5 × 2.5 × 2.4 meter chamber for 4 hr during moderate exercise. Eighteen hours later the subjects underwent bronchoscopy, which included bronchial lavage and bronchial biopsy to evaluate biochemical and morphological changes. The study was done carefully and a number of end points were examined, including pulmonary function. None of the assessments of respiratory toxicity showed any effects from HNO_3 gas in the 10 subjects. Therefore, a human no-observed-effect level (NOEL) for HNO_3 can be established as 0.2 ppm for 4 hr.

Other investigators have tested lower concentrations of HNO_3 on human subjects. Becker et al. (1992) showed that a 200-µg/m³ (0.08 ppm) exposure for 2 hr produced no adverse respiratory effects in nine human subjects. That concentration was chosen to represent a concentration of HNO_3 that was higher than those observed in ambient air (EPA 1993); ambient concentrations ranged from 0.1 to 20 ppb. Later, Becker et al. (1996) used the same exposure concentration and duration, but did not observe any adverse effects as judged by bronchoalveolar lavage and pulmonary-function tests. None of the biochemical measures, such as protein levels, lactate dehydrogenase (LDH), and fibronectin, changed as a result of the exposure. The investigators observed a surprising increase in the phagocytic activity of alveolar macrophages from exposed individuals, but that was not believed to be an adverse effect. Therefore, no toxic effects occurred in humans exposed to HNO_3 for 2 hr at 0.08 ppm.

The use of a 0.2-ppm NOEL for healthy humans exposed to HNO_3 based on the study of Aris et al. (1993) appears appropriate. However, the studies of Koenig et al. (1989a,b) indicate that individuals with asthma might be more sensitive than those without. In these studies, adolescent asthmatic subjects (six males and nine females) with exercise-induced bronchospasm were exposed via a rubber mouthpiece with nose clips to HNO_3 aerosol at a concentration of 0.05 ppm (130 µg/m³). Respiratory function was measured at the end of the exposure. The exposure at 0.05 ppm for 40 min (30 min at rest followed by a 10-min moderate exercise period) produced a decrease in forced expiratory volume (FEV) of 4% and an increase in respiratory resistance of 23% (Koenig et al. 1989a). The authors concluded that individuals with asthma represent a population group that might be exquisitely more sensitive to the effects of HNO_3 than healthy individuals.

However, another study of allergic adolescents selected by the same criteria (Koenig et al. 1989b) showed no effect at the same exposure concentration of HNO_3 for 45 min with 2 15-min moderate exercise periods and a 15-min rest period between exercise periods. The results of that study are different from those of the previous investigation in that no changes in respiratory function were produced, despite the increased period of exercise during the exposure. However, the exercise rate, measured as volume of air expired per minute, was slightly lower in the second study (Koenig et al. 1989b), 25 L/min, than in the first study (Koenig et al. 1989a), 32 L/min. The authors attempted to explain the lack of an effect in the second study by emphasizing that the two studies were conducted during different parts of the calendar year. However, it is difficult to rationalize why testing in summer months would produce effects and testing in winter months would not produce effects in a well-controlled study, because cold-induced bronchospasm often occurs in those with asthma. The subcommittee concludes that, although the results of the two human studies appear to be contradictory, exposure to HNO_3 at 0.05 ppm for 40 to 45 min might cause respiratory problems in certain sensitive subgroups such as in asthmatic individuals. That low exposure concentration and duration can be used to establish a NOEL for the subgroup of asthmatic individuals in the general population.

Table F-1 summarizes the quantitative exposure-response data for humans exposed to HNO_3 via inhalation.

EFFECTS IN ANIMALS

Only a few studies have been conducted in which animals have been exposed to HNO_3 via inhalation. HNO_3 was administered via instillation in a number of studies, but that protocol represents an artificial method of administering HNO_3 directly to the respiratory tract. Although the method provides a good determination of the toxicities of

TABLE F-1 Summary of Exposure-Response Data for HNO_3

Species, no.	Exposure Duration	Exposure Concentration $\mu g/m^3$	Exposure Concentration ppm[1]	Effect Concentration, ppm	End Points	References
Human (12) (asthmatic)	3 min	40,000	15	15	Broncho-constriction	Balmes et al. 1989
Human (10)	4 hr	500	0.2	—	No change in pulmonary function or BAL	Aris et al. 1993
Human (9)	2 hr	200	0.08	—	No change in airway resistance or inflammation (BAL)	Becker et al. 1992
Human (9)	2 hr	200	0.08	—	No change in pulmonary function	Becker et al. 1996
Human (9) (asthmatic)	40 min	129	0.05	0.05	FEV decreased by 4%; respiratory resistance increased by 23%	Koenig et al. 1989a
Human (9) (asthmatic)	45 min total: 15 min, exercise; 15 min, rest; 15 min, exercise	126	0.05	—	No change in FEV and respiratory resistance	Koenig et al. 1989b
Sheep (healthy and allergic)	4 hr	4,120	1.6	1.6	Decreased pulmonary resistance	Abraham et al. 1982
Rat	4 hr	644, 2,575	0.251	0.25	Reduction in respiratory burst of macrophages	Nadziejko et al. 1992

[1]The term "ppm" is appropriate for gaseous HNO_3, not acidic aerosols, because dissociation of the acid would occur in water vapor. However, for this table and associated text, ppm is used for exposures to aerosols as well as exposures to gaseous HNO_3.

Abbreviations: BAL, bronchoalveolar lavage; FEV, forced expiratory volume.

HNO₃ to tissues along the respiratory tract, the relevance of that method of administration is certainly questionable for human exposures to clouds of combustion products that contain HNO_3. Thus, installation studies will not be used to evaluate inhalation exposure-response levels in this report. Therefore, only two studies are listed in Table F-1, and both of those studies exposed sheep and rats to HNO_3 vapor.

Abraham et al. (1982) exposed seven healthy sheep and seven allergic sheep to HNO_3 vapor at 1.6 ppm for 4 hr. The seven allergic sheep used in this study were characterized by their response (bronchospasm) to inhalation of a 1:20 dilution of *Ascaris suum* extract antigen. The animals had a mean pulmonary flow resistance of 1.4 ± 0.7 cm of H_2O/mL of lipopolysaccharide (LPS) before the antigen challenge, and 5.8 ± 4.1 cm of H_2O/mL of LPS after the challenge. Two of the healthy sheep had large increases in air reactivity after HNO_3 exposure; increases of over 100% in specific airway resistance of the lung occurred after carbachol challenge. Effects in the allergic sheep were more pronounced than in the nonallergic sheep. Nadziejko et al. (1992) observed a reduction in the ability of macrophages to generate a burst of superoxide in rats exposed to vapors of HNO_3 at 0.25 ppm for 4 hr.

The work of Abraham et al. (1982) with sheep and the studies of Nadziejko et al. (1992) with rats established the respiratory toxicity of HNO_3 vapor exposures in animals. These studies show that 1.6 ppm is the lowest-observable-effect level (LOEL) for decreased pulmonary resistance in sheep and 0.25 ppm is the LOEL for reduction in respiratory burst of macrophages in rats. The reduction in respiratory burst of macrophages in rats is probably not an appropriate end point for setting a no-effect human exposure level, especially if uncertainty factors are applied to that level (see "Evaluation of Toxicity Information"), because reduction in macrophage function is not necessarily predictive of an adverse response in animals or humans. Conversely, HNO_3 administration to sheep caused increased pulmonary resistance, and the subcommittee considers that a moderate adverse effect. In the sheep study, allergic sheep were slightly more sensitive to HNO_3 exposures than healthy sheep.

ESTABLISHED INHALATION EXPOSURE LIMITS

Table F-2 summarizes established inhalation exposure limits for HNO_3. ACGIH set the Threshold Limit Value (TLV) time-weighted average

TABLE F-2 Currently Recommended Exposure Limits for Nitric Acid

Exposure Limit	Concentration	Reference
ACGIH TLV-TWA	2 ppm (5.2 mg/m3)	ACGIH 1994
OSHA PEL	2 ppm	U.S. Dept. of Labor 1998
NIOSH REL	2 ppm	NIOSH 1994a
ACGIH TLV-STEL	4 ppm ($\approx$ 10 mg/m3)	ACGIH 1994; NIOSH 1994a
NIOSH IDLH	25 ppm	NIOSH 1994b
Level 1	0.033 ppm (0.086 mg/m^3)	Cal EPA 1995

Abbreviations: ACGIH, American Conference of Governmental Industrial Hygienists; TLV, Threshold Limit Value; TWA, time-weighted average; OSHA, Occupational Safety and Health Administration; PEL, permissible exposure level; NIOSH, National Institute for Occupational Safety and Health; REL, recommended exposure limit; STEL, short-term exposure limit; IDLH, immediately dangerous to life and health.

(TWA) for HNO_3 at 2 ppm to be intermediate between the TLV for hydrogen chloride (5 ppm, ceiling) and the TLV for sulfuric acid (0.25 ppm). The TLV-short-term exposure limit is twice the TLV-TWA value.

EVALUATION OF TOXICITY INFORMATION

Effects from exposures to HNO_3 can range from severe to mild, depending on exposure concentration; however, the relation between exposure concentration, duration, and severity of effect has not been quantified. Inhalation of aerosols or vapors of HNO_3 can produce severe edema and result in death in humans, but the exposure concentrations associated with death are very high and have not been measured. Mild effects resulting from exposure to HNO_3 include temporary nasal and eye irritation, which are common responses to acids. Other mild effects could include the reduction of respiratory burst of macrophages that have been observed in animals. Moderate effects include reductions in respiratory function, sometimes associated with bronchoconstriction. Those effects have been demonstrated almost exclusively in sensitive human populations (those with asthma). The data on HNO_3 toxicity are too few to allow estimation of a dose-response function for any health end point. Some data might be used to estimate exposure concentrations and durations at which no adverse health effects would be expected in exposed human populations.

If the study on rats by Nadziejko et al. (1992) were used to estimate a no-effect level for humans, applying an uncertainty factor of 10 to estimate a NOEL from a LOEL and an uncertainty factor of 10 to estimate effects in humans from effects in rats would yield a no-effect level of 0.0025 ppm in humans. However, as is demonstrated by the work of Aris et al. (1993), that level is far below the no-effect level for healthy humans. The subcommittee concludes, therefore, that changes in macrophage function in rats caused by this chemical are not an appropriate end point for predicting no-effect levels for the respiratory effects of HNO_3 in humans.

If a LOEL-to-NOEL uncertainty factor of 10 and an animal-to-human uncertainty factor of 10 are applied to the 1.6 ppm effect level for a 4-hr exposure of sheep from the work of Abraham et al. (1982), a value of 0.016 ppm is predicted to be a no-effect level in humans. That value is more than a factor of 10 below the observed no-effect level in human studies and would be more conservative than necessary to protect healthy humans.

The study by Aris et al. (1993) identified a NOEL for exposure of healthy humans to HNO_3 at 0.2 ppm for a period of 4 hr. To establish a NOEL for periods of 1 hr or less, Haber's rule is used to extrapolate from 0.2 ppm at 4 hr to a NOEL of 1.0 ppm (0.8 ppm rounded up) for a period of 1 hr or less. Haber's rule states that the biological effects of some types of inhalation toxicants are related to the total cumulative exposure, that is the time-weighted-average concentration multiplied by the duration of exposure. Given that acute HNO_3-induced inhalation toxicity results from the corrosive or acidic nature of the compound in the respiratory tract, Haber's rule is expected to apply to this compound over relatively short exposure durations. The subcommittee considers that exposure concentration to be a ceiling value, because toxicity can be observed in humans at concentrations about 15 times higher than 0.2 ppm for a short period. In addition, concentrations substantially higher that 1.0 ppm might produce decreased pulmonary resistance in humans, effects similar to those seen at 1.6 ppm in sheep.

The studies with human asthmatic subjects have shown that this portion of the population might be more sensitive to HNO_3 than healthy individuals. As discussed above, the two studies by Koenig et al. (1989a,b) provide somewhat different results but suggest that some asthmatic individuals under some conditions might experience a mild, reversible increase in respiratory resistance when exposed to HNO_3 at concentrations as low as 0.05 ppm. Therefore, the subcommittee believes that 0.05 ppm should be considered a ceiling value for HNO_3 exposure of humans with compromised respiratory function.

RESEARCH NEEDS

It is obvious from the discussion above that a major research need for HNO_3 is to establish exposure-response information in animals or humans. The concentrations that produce no effects in humans are well founded, but an important gap exists in the exposure-response data between the 0.2-ppm NOEL and the 15-ppm concentration that produces bronchoconstriction. In addition, including sensitive individuals (e.g., with asthma) in the same experiment would be valuable in defining their relative sensitivity. A carefully performed study on experimental animals that includes a wide range of doses and functional, as well as histopathological, end points could be used to establish an exposure-response function for this chemical.

REFERENCES

Abraham, W.M., C.S. Kim, M.M. King, W. Oliver, Jr., and L. Yerger. 1982. Effects of HNO_3 on carbochol reactivity of the airways in normal and allergic sheep. Arch. Environ. Health 37:36-40.

ACGIH (American Conference of Governmental Industrial Hygienists). 1994. 1994-1995 Threshold Limit Values for Chemical Substances and Physical Agents and Biological Exposure Indices. American Conference of Governmental Industrial Hygienists, Cincinnati, Ohio.

AIHA (American Industrial Hygiene Association). 1997. Emergency Response Planning Guideline: ERPG Nitric Acid (draft). AIHA Emergency Response Planning Guideline Committee. American Industrial Hygiene Association, Fairfax, Va.

Aris, R., D. Christian, I. Tager, L. Ngo, W.E. Finkbeiner, and J.R. Balmes. 1993. Effects of HNO3 gas alone or in combination with ozone on healthy volunteers. Am. Rev. Respir. Dis. 148:965-973.

Balmes, J.R., J.M. Fine, T. Gordon, and D. Sheppard. 1989. Potential bronchoconstrictor stimuli in acid fog. Environ. Health Perspect. 79:163-166.

Becker, S., L.J. Roger, R.B. Devlin, and H.S. Koren. 1992. Increased phagocytosis and antiviral activity of alveolar macrophages from humans exposed to nitric acid [abstract]. Am. Rev. Resp. Dis. 145:A429.

Becker, S., L.J. Roger, R.B. Devlin, D.H. Horstman, and H.S. Koren. 1996. Exposure to HNO_3 stimulates human alveolar macrophage function but does not cause inflammation or changes in lung function. Inhal. Toxicol. 8:185-200.

Cal EPA (California Environmental Protection Agency). 1995. Technical Support Document for the Determination of Acute Toxicity Exposure Levels for Airborne Toxicants. Draft for Public Comment. Office of Environmental Health Hazard Assessment. January.

EPA (U.S. Environmental Protection Agency). 1982. Air Quality Criteria for Oxides of Nitrogen. EPA/600/8-82-026. U.S. Environmental Protection Agency, Office of Health and Environmental Assessment, Environmental Criteria and Assessment Office, Research Triangle Park, N.C. Available from NTIS, Springfield, Va., Doc. No. PB83-131011.

EPA (U.S. Environmental Protection Agency). 1993. Pp. 7-5, 7-6 in Air Quality Criteria for Oxides of Nitrogen, Vol. 1. EPA/600/8-91/049aF. U.S. Environmental Protection Agency, Washington, D.C.

Gosselin, R.E., R.P. Smith, and H.C. Hodge. 1984. Clinical Toxicology of Commercial Products, 5th Ed. Baltimore, Md.: Williams & Wilkins.

Hajela, R., D.T. Janigan, P.L. Landrigan, S.F. Boudreau, and S. Sebastian. 1990. Fatal pulmonary edema due to nitric acid fume inhalation in three pulp-mill workers. Chest 97:487-489.

Koenig, J.Q., D.S. Covert, and W.E. Pierson. 1989a. Effects of inhalation of acidic compounds on pulmonary function in allergic adolescent subjects. Environ. Health Perspect. 79:173-178.

Koenig, J.Q., Q.S. Hanley, T.L. Anderson, V. Rebolledo, and W.E. Pierson. 1989b. An Assessment of Pulmonary Function Changes and Oral Ammonia Levels after Exposure of Adolescent Asthmatic Subjects to Sulfuric or Nitric Acid. Abstract 89-92.4 in Proceedings of the 82nd Annual Meeting of the Air & Waste Management Association. Pittsburgh, Pa.: Air & Waste Management Association.

Lioy, P.J., and M. Lippmann. 1986. Measurement of exposure to acidic sulfur aerosols. Pp. 743-752 in Aerosols, S.D. Lee and T. Schneider, eds. Chelsea, Mich.: Lewis.

Lippmann, M. 1989a. Background on health effects of acid aerosols. Environ. Health Perspect. 79:3-6.

Lippmann, M. 1989b. Progress, prospects, and research needs on the health effects of acid aerosols. Environ. Health Perspect. 79:203-205.

Nadziejko, C.E., L. Nansen, R.C. Mannix, M.T. Kleinman, and R.F. Phalen. 1992. The effect of nitric acid vapor on the response to inhaled ozone. Inhal. Toxicol. 4:343-358.

NIOSH (National Institute of Occupational Safety and Health). 1994a. NIOSH Pocket Guide to Chemical Hazards. NIOSH Publ. No. 94-116. National Institute of Occupational Safety and Health, Cincinnati, Ohio.

NIOSH (National Institute for Occupational Safety and Health). 1994b. Documentation for Immediately Dangerous to Life or Health Concentrations (IDLHs). NIOSH Division of Standards, Development and Technology Transfer, Cincinnati, Ohio. Available from NTIS, Springfield, Va., Doc. No. PB94-195047.

U.S. Department of Labor. 1998. Occupational Safety and Health Standards. Air Contaminants. Title 29, Code of Federal Regulations, Part 1910, Section 1910.1000. Washington, D.C.: U.S. Government Printing Office.

Wolff, G.T., M.S. Ruthkosky, D.P. Stroup, and P.E. Korsog. 1991. A characterization of the principal PM-10 species in Claremont (summer) and Long Beach (fall) during SCAQS. Atmos. Environ. Part A 25:2173-2186.